In Her Shoes:

DANCING IN THE SHADOW OF CANCER

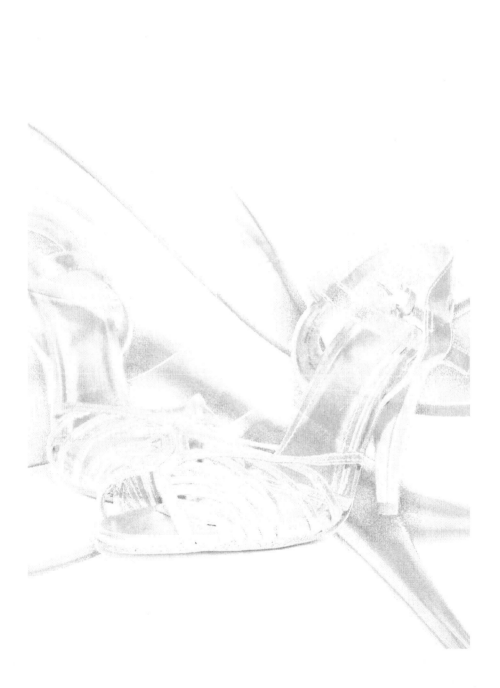

Endorsements

Author Joanie Shawhan, a former oncology nurse, shares snippets from her own cancer journey and experiences from others to give an honest portrayal of the scares, heartaches, and pains of the disease. However, she doesn't stop there. She adds comforting, hope-filled Bible verses and prayers to each chapter, and she sprinkles helpful hints and practical advice throughout. As a survivor myself, I know that dancing in the shadow of cancer isn't easy, but it *is* possible. Reading this book is a good first step.

—**Twila Belk**. Writer, speaker, and author of *The Power to Be: Be Still, Be Grateful, Be Strong, Be Courageous* and *Raindrops from Heaven: Gentle Reminders of God's Power, Presence, and Purpose.*

Joanie Shawhan has written a down-to-earth book about cancer, *In Her Shoes: Dancing in the Shadow of Cancer.* The cancer patient will receive comfort, compassion, and a companion in Joanie Shawhan. The author guides not only the cancer patient but also family and friends. She has been where they are now, and she understands. I highly recommend this book.

—**Yvonne Ortega**, LPC. (Licensed Professional Counselor), cancer survivor, and author of *Moving from Broken to Beautiful® through Grief*

If cancer came knocking on your door, *In Her Shoes: Dancing in the Shadow of Cancer* will offer you the hand of a friend. Through her own story, Joanie invites the reader to come along on her journey through and out of ovarian cancer. The vignettes of other survivors in the second half of the book add to the big picture of courage and hope. I will recommend this book to both patients and practitioners.

—**Letitia Suk**, author of *Getaway with God.*

In her book, *In Her Shoes: Dancing in the Shadow of Cancer,* Joanie Shawhan shares her inspirational and heartfelt personal journey as an ovarian cancer survivor. Through her courageous experiences and the stories shared by other survivors, Joanie offers readers a very real glimpse of what is endured throughout a cancer diagnosis. This book is a must read for all survivors, caregivers, and those with a loved one currently fighting.

—**Ashley Wagner**, Executive Director Wisconsin Ovarian Cancer Alliance

Joanie Shawhan has courageously written about her own trials through ovarian cancer treatment so others can find solace and hope. I highly encourage my fellow pastors, church leaders, counselors, friends and family to give this book to any woman who has been told she has ovarian cancer. Reading this book will draw each woman closer to God while giving her practical survival tips. But this book is also for those who walk alongside these brave women because it depicts an honest description of what happens to the body, the soul, and the spirit of those we love during their journey. Thank you, Joanie, for sharing your story, your wisdom, and your prayers.

—**Tess Brunmeier**, MA Psychological Counseling, M.Div. Regent University, Lead pastor of Covenant Community Fellowship, New Albany, IN.

In Her Shoes: Dancing in the Shadow of Cancer was inspirational. The author shares tragic and sometimes humorous experiences. The book is a wonderful resource for those making the journey of cancer treatment and recovery. It would also be an informative and motivating story for nursing students or novice oncology nurses. As a nurse and as a woman, I found myself reflecting on my role and my responsibilities to patients and friends struggling with cancer treatment. I would recommend this book for anyone touched by cancer.

—**Molly Cluskey**, Ph.D. RN, CNE; Associate Dean, Distance Education, College of Education and Health Sciences, Bradley University, Peoria, IL.

In Her Shoes:

Dancing in the Shadow of Cancer

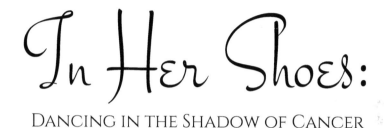

Joanie Shawhan

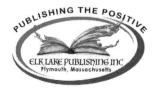

PUBLISHING THE POSITIVE

ELK LAKE PUBLISHING INC.
Plymouth, Massachusetts

Library Cataloging Data

Names: Shawhan, Joanie (Joanie Shawhan)

In Her Shoes: Dancing in the Shadow of Cancer / Joanie Shawhan

302 p. 23cm × 15cm (9in × 6 in.)

Description: Stories of women who have been victorious in their battles against various kinds of cancer.

Identifiers: ISBN-13: 978-1-950051-18-2 (trade) | 978-1-950051-19-9 (POD)

| 978-1-950051-20-5 (e-book.)

Key Words: Breast cancer, ovarian cancer, leukemia, brain cancer, inspirational, women's issues

Dedication

I dedicate *In Her Shoes: Dancing in the Shadow of Cancer* to the memory of my sister, Tracy, who courageously battled cancer and to all those who have fought or are fighting this disease.

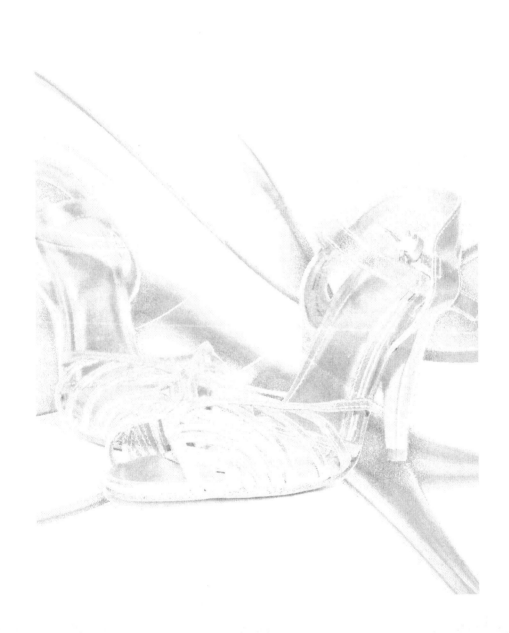

Acknowledgments

I send my gratitude to my family, friends and health care providers who walked with me through my battle with cancer. Thank you to those in the publishing industry and my fellow writers who taught me how to write and mentored me on this writing journey. I want to especially thank the following:

Mom (Luella Shawhan) who stayed with me throughout my surgery and prayed for me. You opened the door for me to the world of books. When the flyer for books arrived from my school, you always purchased my requested stack.

My sisters Jean and Kate who were also by my side during surgery. Thank you, Jean, for showing me that hats and scarves can be fun.

My physicians. Thank you to my gynecologist, Dr. Linda Neidhart, for your care and compassion throughout my diagnosis, surgery, and follow-up. Dr. Michael Frontiera—without your kindness and support I would never have made it through my chemotherapy treatments.

My intercessory prayer team. Thank you, Dennis and Kathy Rinzel, Kathy Shafarik, Stephen Gill, Mary Gill, and Ann Sippy. We have laughed, cried, prayed, and done life together. I cannot express how much all of your love, prayers, and support through the years mean to me. Thank you Susan (Spanky) Lloyd, Julie Shephard, and Pastor Bryan and Debbie Peterson for praying for me and coming to my aid.

My fellow contributors. Thank you for so graciously sharing your cancer journeys with me: Anna, Cathie, Jill, Joanne, Lisa, Pat, Rita, Ruth, Stacy, Sue, and Val. Your stories will encourage many women and their loved ones whose lives have been affected by cancer.

Barnes and Noble and The Middleton Library. Thank you for providing me alternative writing haunts.

Support networks. I want to thank the groups and organizations that taught me to thrive: Camp Mak-A-Dream, the YMCA's Livestrong program, The Wisconsin Ovarian Cancer Alliance (WOCA), and The Fried Eggs—Sunny Side Up.

IN HER SHOES: DANCING IN THE SHADOW OF CANCER

Friends of the Pen. I have learned so much from each one of you as we have shared our writing journeys together. Anita Klumpers, Lori Lipsky, Sue Smith, and Robin Steinweg, you have shaped me into a better writer.

WordGirls. I am so grateful for each of you in this writing community mentored by Kathy Carlton Willis where we have grown as writers, prayed, and encouraged one another.

Michelle Rayburn. Thank you for your thorough attention to detail in formatting and editing my manuscript to Elk Lake Publishing standards.

Kathy Carlton Willis. I cannot thank you enough for the mentoring, teaching, encouragement, brainstorming, networking, and wisdom you have so generously poured into me. When I was overwhelmed, you broke my project down into smaller goals so I could accomplish them one step at a time.

Deb Haggerty and Elk Lake Publishing. I am so grateful that *In Her Shoes: Dancing in the Shadow of Cancer* is a book you also envisioned. Thank you for publishing my project. Thank you, Derinda Babcock, for designing such a beautiful book cover. I loved it from the moment I first saw your design.

Jeanne Leach. I am so thankful that Deb at Elk Lake Publishing selected you to be my editor. I felt an instant rapport with you and I so enjoyed working with you. Thank you for your encouragement, support, and teaching moments.

Diana Flegal and Hartline Literary Agency. Thank you catching the vision for *In Her Shoes: Dancing in the Shadow of Cancer* and representing me.

Our Lord Jesus Christ. You lovingly navigated me through this cancer storm and opened doors for me I never could have imagined. I dedicate this book to your glory.

Table of Contents

Introduction

Why I Wrote *In Her Shoes: Dancing in the Shadow of Cancer*

When the doctor pronounced my diagnosis of ovarian cancer, I was shocked. We had agreed the tumor was a fibroid. Numb, I went through the motions of more tests and consultations with the surgery and oncology teams. As a nurse with an oncology background, I should have been equipped with the knowledge I needed to cope with cancer, but I had more questions than answers. Where could I go for more information, support, and camaraderie?

My oncologist patiently explained my prognosis, treatment, and side effects. His words emanated a kindness, so opposite the harsh treatment I would receive. My friend Jill, who survived a childhood cancer, told me about the "Look Good Feel Better" program that provided wigs and makeup tips through the American Cancer Society. This organization also sent me information on ovarian cancer and chemotherapy.

But where were the other ovarian cancer survivors? Were there others? Did they not live long enough to form support groups like breast cancer survivors? Even though I had wonderful friends and prayer support, I missed having the opportunity to share my journey with other cancer survivors, to learn from their stories, and to validate my own experiences.

Cancer is hard. For me, the treatment was even worse than the symptoms caused by the cancer itself. Even though my oncologist explained the side effects, I wasn't prepared for total body demolition. By trial and error, I learned how to cope with the side effects as each round of chemotherapy left me increasingly debilitated.

As I chronicled my recovery, I found I had a voice and a message that could help other women navigating cancer and its treatment. My writing focused on individual aspects of my journey, concluding each vignette with a Scripture and a prayer.

Later, I realized there were other women with their own unique cancer stories waiting to be shared—everyday women with everyday lives interrupted by cancer. Since their experiences were different from mine, I wanted to include their stories to make *In Her Shoes: Dancing in the Shadow of Cancer* relatable to more women. The purpose of this book is not to focus on *my* story but about coming alongside others with the help I desired when I went through my treatment.

I lost my identity to ovarian cancer. Who was I as a woman? Hairless, and my female parts gutted, I languished on a couch instead of nursing my patients back to health.

But after I recovered, I discovered a new purpose and a new calling in my life—to write encouraging articles for women undergoing chemotherapy and to advocate for and educate women regarding ovarian cancer.

I pray you will identify with these stories and leave the pages of *In Her Shoes: Dancing in the Shadow of Cancer* feeling validated, encouraged, and filled with hope.

In a dance not of my own choosing, the Lord extended his hand—a hand of grace, blessings, and comfort throughout my personal battle. I wish to offer this same hope to my readers so they too may dance in the shadow of cancer.

The Other Side of the Bed

I was no stranger to the ravages of chemotherapy. I had devoted six years to oncology nursing. We stimulated immune systems and heated, poisoned, targeted, and irradiated cancer cells. Our treatments blasted unsuspecting bodies while we managed the side effects: rigors, headaches, infections, fatigue, nausea, and pain. We slathered inflamed, irradiated skin with soothing cream. Before our patients nibbled on soft, bland food, we coated their ulcerated mouths with numbing gel. Sallow skin sagged over their brittle bones as our desperate patients picked at their macrobiotic diets. Between controlling their pain and brushing wisps of hair away from feverish brows, we cradled their frail hands.

My personal battle with ovarian cancer triggered memories of these past patients—the courageous warriors with whom we laughed and cried. We shared their families, their hopes, their dreams, and even their holidays. We grieved during their setbacks and rejoiced with their victories. Sometimes, I feared our treatment would kill them before eradicating the cancer.

In light of this, I vowed to never undergo chemotherapy. But now, I felt powerless to carry out this resolution. I was one of them, dragged through the theme park of cancer, only I hadn't purchased a ticket. Clapping my hands over my ears, I attempted to block the call of the barker as he beckoned me into a game of roulette—my life the prize. The tune "What If?" revolved around my mind like a crazed carousel. How I yearned to grasp the switch that would halt this fearsome ride. But if I wanted to live, I needed to go forward with the treatment.

Cancer flung me to the other side of the bed. Nursing scrubs and shoes gave way to tieback gowns and skid-free gripper socks. Instead of my fingers threading needles into sunken veins, other nurses laced the sharp tips into my veins. Malaise, pain, and nausea stormed my body. The side effects I now managed were my own.

Despite the onslaught of cancer and chemotherapy, I felt reassured that I had made the right decision. I pressed forward. But I often questioned God. In times of prayer, and with his Word and his peace, he ushered me through the fears of all that could go wrong, the chemotherapy that pummeled me, and the voices that spewed negativity.

Several months later, I once again donned my nursing scrubs and resumed my career on the other side of the bed. God had guided me safely through the maze of cancer and chemotherapy.

> For this God is our God for ever and ever; he will be our guide
> even to the end. (Psalm 48:14 NIV)

Prayer: Lord, thank you for taking my hand and leading me through this difficult season. Through your faithfulness, you have brought me out on the other side.

Part 1

My Story

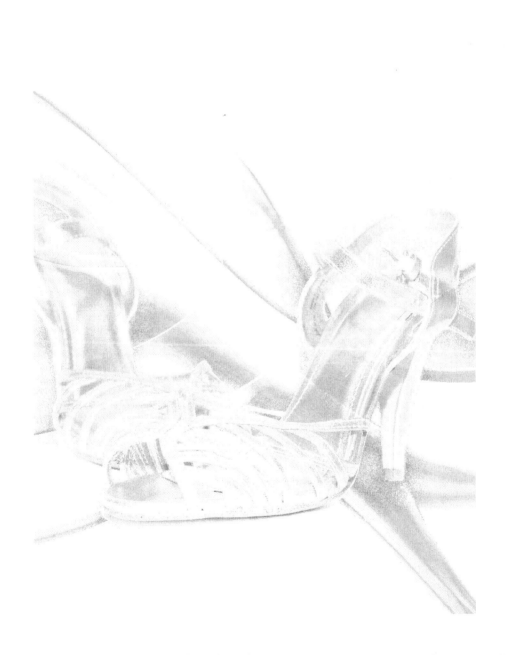

Chapter 1

A Rude Awakening

Groggy from sleep, I rolled over in bed, compressing a hard lump in my abdomen. My eyes flew open, adjusting to the darkness that shrouded the room. I clutched the grapefruit-sized mass. My heart thumped. Questions popped into my head like the pings and alarms of a pinball machine. What is this hard bulge? Will I need surgery? Can I still go on my mission trip to India? Maybe this bump would just disappear, a bad dream spawned by an overactive imagination.

Several days later, I lay prone on a physical therapy table for an evaluation of a recent back injury that occurred at work. With a firm, even pressure, the physical therapist walked his fingers down either side of my spine. When he reached my lower back, I tensed and cried out in excruciating pain. But my back was not the culprit. Pain had shot through my abdomen and confirmed my worst fears—something was very wrong.

The therapist removed his hands from my back and assisted me to a sitting position. I pressed my hands on the table to stop them from shaking and quell the dizziness before I stood. We agreed to postpone any further evaluation of my back injury.

Twenty minutes later, I sped across town, praying my friend Kathy would be home. Kathy answered the door and suggested we sit out in her backyard. We settled onto the picnic benches in the privacy of her gardens, still flourishing beneath the Indian summer sun. I tried to calm my racing heart, but a mounting fear squeezed my chest like a boa constrictor. I couldn't speak quickly enough as I recounted my physical therapy visit and my abdominal mass.

Kathy walked back into the house and returned with a telephone directory and the phone.

With trembling hands, I flipped through the pages, located the doctor's number, and dialed.

"I have a mass in my abdomen," I said to the receptionist.

"Let me check the schedule and see when I can get you an appointment with the doctor," she replied.

I pressed the phone to my ear. Silence. My stomach tightened as I strained to hear her voice again.

"I have an appointment available at the end of next week."

"I'll take it."

I waited. I prayed. I hoped.

Wait for the LORD; be strong and take heart and wait for the LORD. (Psalm 27:14 NIV)

Prayer: Lord, as I wait for answers, I also wait for direction from you. Thank you for strengthening me during this season of waiting.

Chapter 2

The Verdict

My knees quivered to the rhythm of my pounding heart as the nurse led me into the exam room of a doctor I had never met. I settled in the chair and prayed while I waited. Deep breath, slowly exhale, and repeat.

Fifteen minutes later, I heard a knock on the door. The doctor slid the door open and introduced herself, disarming me with her smile. We discussed my medical history which included surgery for endometriosis twenty years prior to the arrival of this new abdominal mass. I climbed onto the exam table, and she performed her physical exam.

"Could this be just a fibroid?" I cautiously asked my doctor. "Will I still be able to go on my mission trip to India in two months?"

"A fibroid is quite probable," she reassured me. "It's about the size of a cantaloupe, but we'll need to do an ultrasound just to be sure. As long as you're not too uncomfortable, India shouldn't be a problem."

As I exited the office, I felt the tension ease off my shoulders like a drained battery in a tightly wound toy.

The following week, I arrived at my ultrasound appointment—alone. I'd reassured my friends I would be okay. After all, it was just a fibroid, right? As the technician explained the procedure, she smeared the cold ultrasound gel on my abdomen. The remote screen emitted the only light in that darkened room. Pressing the probe on my abdomen, she slid the instrument back and forth. Her brow furrowed. She shot me a glance. Something was wrong.

The technician slipped the films into an oversize envelope and instructed me to deliver them to the receptionist upstairs. We had scheduled my doctor appointment immediately following the ultrasound.

I tucked the ultrasound films under my arm, barreled through the crowded waiting room, and deposited them into the receptionist's outstretched hand.

She directed me to take a seat. I sought out a quiet corner, but I could find no relief from the voices screaming in my mind—something's wrong. I perched on the edge of my chair and drummed my fingers on the wooden armrests. How I wished I hadn't been so hasty in my decision to come alone. I crossed and uncrossed my legs, bounced my foot, and reassured myself that I had certainly misinterpreted the technician's reaction. *Please, God, let me have misinterpreted her expression.*

A technician ushered me into the exam room. I stared at the gray table spread with its dull, white paper, torn at the edges, and waited.

The doctor strode in. The words "probable ovarian cancer" rolled off her tongue. In the same breath, she rattled off tests that needed to be done immediately: labs for the ovarian cancer marker and liver studies, CT scan of my abdomen and pelvis, a mammogram, and surgery scheduled at first availability.

The technician led me out of the exam room and into the surgery scheduling office. Surgical dates spewed from the scheduler's lips until I latched onto one less than two weeks away. Numb, I went through the motions of lab draws and test schedules. Anxiety intermingled with the details and whipped around my mind like a blender at high-speed. Between juggling my test appointments, I attempted to phone my family and friends. But each time, a voice recording answered my silent scream for help.

Finally, I reached one of my India team members. "I have cancer. I'm still at the clinic. The doctor ordered a CT scan which I'll have this afternoon."

"Oh, Joanie! I'm so sorry. Would you like me to come and sit with you?"

"Yes." Tears pooled in my eyes. My friend had offered to leave work just to be with me.

We sat in the radiology waiting room. She distracted me with our plans for India while I sipped on the chalky-berry CT contrast.

The tech ushered me into the CT scanner and instructed me to lie down on the cold, hard table, facing the hollow cylinder. She inserted an IV and attached the automated dye syringe. "Try to hold still during the scan. It only takes a few minutes. Just follow the computerized voice instructions," she said. "The dye can cause you to feel flushed, but that's normal."

The table slid me into the scanner's mouth. The scan commenced. The voice instructed me to hold my breath, then exhale. My insides quivered. I hoped the quivering wouldn't interfere with holding myself still.

I continued to work and robotically go through the motions of daily life while I waited for the test results. My stomach churned to the tune of *Please don't let it be cancer.* I wavered between denial and fear. Like crashing waves, the torrents of anxiety overwhelmed me. I cried out to the Lord, but I received no benign reassurances. He reminded me that no matter what my tests revealed, I wouldn't be walking through this ordeal alone. He would be with me.

One week later, I arrived at the doctor's office to receive my test results. My heart raced, pounding against my shallow breaths. I glanced around the room. Swollen bellies heralded new life while my life dangled on a thread.

The nurse called my name and led me to the exam room. "The doctor will be in shortly."

I crossed and uncrossed my legs, scanned the gynecological charts, anatomical models, and informational brochures.

My doctor knocked on the door and strode in. "Your Ca125, the tumor marker for ovarian cancer, is 280. Normal is less than 35," she said. "Your CT scan shows a large mass encompassing your uterus and remaining ovary." She pointed to the mass on the film. "I'm not seeing any spreading to your liver or your lymph nodes. Your liver function tests are normal. We'll know how extensive the cancer is after surgery. Since I'm not an oncology surgeon, our surgical scheduler will schedule surgery with me as well as our gynecologic oncology surgeon."

"Are you sure it's ovarian cancer?" I didn't want to believe her. I couldn't believe her—my façade of control might shatter.

"Yes."

The verdict—ovarian cancer. The sentence—exploratory surgery with a total abdominal hysterectomy in ten days.

> When you pass through the waters, I will be with you; and when you pass through the rivers, they will not sweep over you. When you walk through the fire, you will not be burned; the flames will not set you ablaze. (Isaiah 43:2 NIV)

Prayer: Lord, when I am overwhelmed and afraid, help me to remember you are with me, and I am never alone. Thank you that you will walk with me through everything I face.

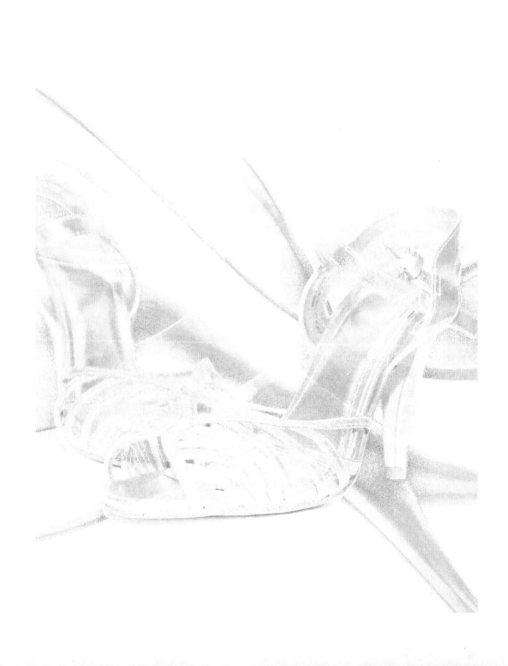

Chapter 3

HELPFUL HINTS:
SO ... YOU HAVE CANCER—NOW WHAT?

1, Ask your doctor what additional tests are needed: pulmonary, heart, genetic or lab; x-rays, scans, MRI, dental, ear or eye exams; biopsies. Are there special instructions you need to follow beforehand?

2. What will your treatment plan include: surgery, medications, chemotherapy, radiotherapy? How often and over what duration?

3. What are the side effects and how will they be managed? Some side effects may extend beyond treatment.

4. Are there any medical restrictions: food, medications, supplements, activity?

5. Supply your doctor with a list of your current medications including over-the-counter and herbal supplements.

6. Be sure to tell your doctor if you have any food, medication, or latex allergies.

7. Write down any questions you may have and bring this list to your doctor. Bring a small notebook and pen to jot down the answers to questions and any new information. A diagnosis of cancer can be overwhelming, and you may not remember all that was said during the visit. Some find it helpful to bring a friend to take notes.

8. What type of follow-up can you expect: scans, labs including tumor markers, further biopsies? At what intervals and duration?

9. Ask your provider about what other resources may be available to you such as: social worker, nutritional consultation, psychologist, physical and occupational therapy. Request a resource list.

Chapter 4

UNDER THE KNIFE

Faster and faster, the treadmill in my brain accelerated. I clamped my hands over my head, willing my mind to remember all of the details. A whirlwind of activity had caught me in its vortex. I notified family, friends, work, and insurance. I cleaned, packed, canceled, and rescheduled. Although I was loved, prayed with, supported, and encouraged, I still was not ready. Is anyone ever truly ready for cancer surgery?

My mom and two of my sisters drove in from Illinois the day before surgery. My required bowel prep squelched any plans for a nice, relaxing dinner. The next morning, darkness mingled with the crispness of fall as we weaved along the deserted streets to the hospital, my sister at the wheel.

In the holding area, I relinquished all of my personal possessions in exchange for a designer hospital gown and compression stockings.

My family, several friends, and my pastor gathered around my bed in the surgical holding area to pray. After goodbye hugs and promises of continued prayer, my friends left to go to work.

The anesthesiologist arrived, verified my identity, and completed his work-up. He attempted multiple IV sticks. With each poke, I clenched my fist and grimaced, hoping my family wouldn't notice. A nurse injected my arm with a pre-op hypo. I said goodbye to my family as the staff whisked me out the door to the operating room.

Bright lights hovered over the stainless-steel operating table. I squinted my eyes beneath their glare. Lining the perimeter of the room, trays of shiny instruments lay nestled in sterile green cloths. The odor of antiseptic filled my nostrils. I wrinkled my nose. Drops of medication plopped from the IV suspended above my head. While counting backward from one hundred, my memory faded.

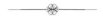

Despite my heavy eyelids, searing abdominal pain jerked me awake in the recovery room. I heard a distant moan. The voice—my own. I pressed the pain button attached to my IV pump. It beeped its consent, and I drifted off to sleep.

Oxygen prongs poked my nostrils. With mounting irritation, I swiped them away, only to find them firmly replaced. My legs felt bathed in ice. I crossed my ankles in hope of kindling some warmth, but the nurse repeatedly uncrossed my legs. Eventually, she draped heated blankets over my shivering form and tucked them around my chilled feet.

Nearby, I heard my doctor's voice discussing surgical results. Was she talking to me? I tried to open my eyes and move my lips, but they felt weighted shut. I registered one word—cancer.

When I awake, I am still with you. (Psalm 139:18 NIV)

Prayer: Thank you, Lord, that no matter what happens in my life, you are always with me. Please help me to trust you when I hear devastating news.

Chapter 5

Go Through the Process

The recovery room staff rolled my bed off the elevator with a clatter. The floor's uneven ledge jostled me. Waves of pain tore through my abdomen. Still groggy, my eyelids slid open as we wheeled past my family huddled nearby with furrowed brows.

Back in my room, I mumbled to my friend Kathy, "It's cancer, right?"

"The doctor didn't think you'd heard what she said," Kathy replied. "Your mom didn't want to be the one to tell you."

That first night passed in a blur as the clicking of my IV pump ticked down the minutes. Like a ship's anchor, drugs weighed down my eyelids. Snatches of conversation encircled my bed. My lips moved to participate, but no words flowed out.

Over the course of the week, family and friends, interspersed with medical personnel, transformed my room into a revolving door. I appreciated their company, a welcome distraction from the doubts and fears that assailed me. The assault of surgery, anemia, and cancer had sapped my strength. Between visitors, I laid the phone alongside the cradle to catch a nap, despite its annoying beep.

Doctors in starched white coats strode in and out with their hands in their pockets, explaining my biopsy results and recommendations for treatment as if they were discussing dinner plans. The benefits and side effects of chemotherapy bombarded my mind: pain, nausea, fatigue, hair loss, and a possible life-threatening allergic reaction.

To distract me, my sister talked up fuzzy hats and paisley scarves while her daughter excitedly surfed the internet for wigs.

A former oncology nurse, I'd vowed I would never receive chemotherapy. I witnessed too many of my patients suffering debilitating side effects. Now,

I confronted my worst nightmare. With a menacing voice, cancer raised its ugly head, pointed its accusing finger and hissed, "You have cancer."

I prayed, discussed my options with family and friends, and weighed the pros and cons of chemotherapy: the side effects, the five-year survival rates, and the medical recommendations. Before I left the hospital, I sensed the Lord whisper, "Go through the process."

> Even though I walk through the darkest valley, I will fear no evil,
> for you are with me. (Psalm 23:4 NIV)

Prayer: Sometimes you ask me to walk through hard places. Thank you, Lord, for walking with me through these times of darkness and for calming my fears.

Chapter 6

EYE TO EYE

The receptionist's fingers raced across the keyboard. The clicking keys echoed in my ears as I answered the computer-generated hospital admission questions. The computer numbered and filed me in cyberspace. The receptionist slapped a band inscribed with my name, birthdate, and hospital ID number around my wrist. With a few cursory instructions and a nod of her head, she directed me to pre-op for cancer surgery.

Our eyes never met.

The next morning after surgery, the resident physician marched into my room with her eyes focused on the open chart in her hands. No "Good morning," or "How are you today?"

She towered over my bed, peeled down my covers, and chided me for removing the plastic compression sleeves from around my legs. The sleeves, meant to prevent blood clots, also prevented me from sleeping as they cyclically inflated and deflated. She tossed her chestnut hair over her shoulder and thrust her cold stethoscope on my tender abdomen.

Her cursory exam completed, she strode out of my room. I don't know the color of her eyes, nor does she know mine.

Later that morning, my surgeon peeked her smiling face around the corner. "How are you doing today?" Her gentle voice melted the icicles that had crystallized in my room during her colleague's visit. Her gaze met mine before she repeated the resident doctor's exam, with a few subtle differences. A hand-warmed stethoscope gently rested on my abdomen. She glanced toward my face to detect the slightest flinch or grimace.

"You're doing great," she said. She paused for questions and to explain what I could expect over the next few days.

These events reminded me that our eyes are often called the windows to the soul, revealing the depths of our emotions. Sometimes our eyes fail to meet due to the distractions of the moment. At other times, we glower our disapproval or rejection. Then, there are those precious moments when we have found approval and acceptance brimming within the eyes of another. I felt validated under my doctor's gaze.

I may feel marginalized by others, crushed by their disapproval, or rejected. But God never disenfranchises me. His eye is always upon me. I am his delight, his beloved.

> Keep me as the apple of your eye; hide me in the shadow of your wings. (Psalm 17:8 NIV)

Prayer: Thank you, Lord, that in the sea of humanity, your eyes of love are always upon me. I never lack significance with you.

Chapter 7

BEAN SOUP

Book in hand, Mom settled in the lounge chair next to my hospital bed, waiting for my final biopsy results. She gazed out the window at the adjacent brick building, rarely turning a page. She'd planned to stay with me for two weeks while I recovered from cancer surgery.

In the evening, she wound her way through several miles of unfamiliar streets back to my apartment alone under the shadows cast by the streetlights. I was afraid she wouldn't eat supper, even though I had offered her leftovers from my well-stocked refrigerator. Instead, she munched on microwave popcorn and stared at the blank television screen. The silence was broken only by the cacophony of questions that bombarded her mind.

One morning, she arrived at the hospital with a spring in her step, all excited about the navy bean soup she had eaten for supper. My friend Ann had surprised her with a hot meal. The bean soup proved to be hearty dinner each night thereafter. By the time I was discharged, the bean soup was nearly gone, but I managed a taste before my mom polished off every serving.

The stress of my surgery had taken a toll on both of us. I was grateful that my mom never had to cook during those two weeks she stayed with me. We received scrumptious meals: soups, lasagna, and baked chicken. But I was most grateful for the pot of bean soup God had provided to warm my mom on those chilly fall evenings.

> He provides you with plenty of food and fills your hearts with joy.
> (Acts 14:17 NIV)

Prayer: Lord, thank you for friends who provide for our loved ones when we are not able to.

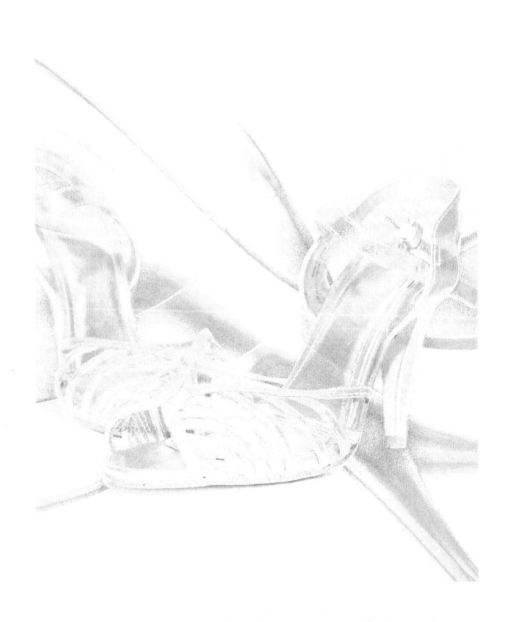

Chapter 8

India Lost

"I think I lost India," I whispered.

I shot a glance toward my friend Julie, with Raggedy Ann painted eyes, perched across from me on Halloween, the day after my surgery. White flowers dotted her navy-blue dress under a white pinafore. Red and white striped stockings peeked out from underneath her white pantaloons. She leaned forward and caressed my hand. Red yarn hair looped around her heart-shaped face. Her eyes filled with tears as she gazed into mine.

"I know," she said.

These two words pierced my heart like a dagger and confirmed what I already knew. I squeezed my eyes shut. I wanted to clap my hands over my ears and shout, "La, la, la, la, la!" at the top of my lungs, but this wouldn't change the awful reality. I wouldn't be able to accompany our team to India for our church mission trip.

India. For over twenty years, these downtrodden people had tugged at my heartstrings. Mother Teresa was my heroine as she scooped the lonely and dying off the streets of Calcutta and demonstrated God's love and compassion to them in their final hours of life.

Nearly two years had passed since a missionary presented the plight of the Dalit people to our church. Our informational session quickly transformed into a planning meeting. The haunting faces of these untouchable, unloved, and unwanted people rekindled my desire for India. We had prayed and set the target date for the following winter when the temperature surge would be hot instead of hottest. Just before the final deadline, our India sponsor canceled our trip due to scheduling conflicts, dashing my hopes and dreams.

We rescheduled our trip for the following winter and were elated as all the details fell into place. The teaching and encouragement from missionaries to India energized us. We had prayed for and sung over the Indian people. We were in the final months of preparation. Airline tickets purchased. Suitcases packed. Vaccinated. Like racehorses, we approached the starting gates, stomped our hooves, and chomped our bits as we awaited the blast of the gun to signal the start of the race.

But chemotherapy held me captive at the gate.

My doctor had crushed any lingering hope of India when he looked deeply into my eyes and said, "You will lack the stamina for such a demanding trip."

Cancer had killed my dream.

> As the heavens are higher than the earth, so are my ways higher than your ways and my thoughts than your thoughts. (Isaiah 55:9 NIV)

Prayer: Lord, I don't understand your timing or your plans, but I choose to trust you.

Chapter 9

LEFT BEHIND?

In a bittersweet farewell, I met with my team the night before they departed for India. I cozied up to the fireplace while we prayed, but even the crackling flames failed to warm my chilled heart. As I hugged each team member goodbye, tears trickled down my cheeks.

Ice had crystallized on my window the morning of their departure. Despite the chill, the Lord woke me with a special gift. He gave me a new song for India, a song to pray and sing over the country's lost and dying people.

That week, I reviewed my journal from the previous year, and I stumbled across an entry regarding our canceled trip to India. I had scrawled, "I have a strange sense of release."

I had forgotten those words, and I didn't understand them at the time. But the Lord knew, even then, that I would be unable to travel to India. He had already released me—yet graciously allowed me to be a part of this dedicated team.

Since I had prepared with the team, I knew their itinerary. I prayed for them as only a fellow team member could. From my rocking chair, I journeyed through India as an intercessor, and toured mission schools where children clad in colorful costumes sang and danced to their traditional music. While vying for attention, orphans laughed and jostled one another.

I visited the Kolar Gold Fields, once a flourishing community but now reduced to a pile of rubble. In exchange for morsels of food, ragged children scoured for trinkets amidst the stench of the garbage dumps. The unemployed scratched the dirt for flecks of gold to eke out a living. Our team erected a movie screen to show the Indian version of a film about Jesus. The life-sized characters lit the night sky.

I remembered the story in the Bible of King David at Ziklag. After a grueling battle where all seemed lost, he proclaimed that those who stayed behind would share in the spoils with those who had gone out to war. Even though I was left behind, God counted India to my credit.

I was not forgotten when our excited, exhausted team returned. They not only shared their stories, pictures, and videos, but also presented me with a paisley shawl from India. Though I never physically stepped foot on Indian soil, I felt honored to be counted as part of the team.

My dreams had lain dashed and shattered against the rocks of life, but the Lord comforted me and caused my heart to dream again. I was not left behind. In my disappointment, I found God's divine appointment.

> When the Lord brought back the captivity of Zion, We were like those who dream. Then our mouth was filled with laughter, And our tongue with singing. Then they said among the nations, "The Lord has done great things for them." (Psalm 126:1-2 NKJV)

Prayer: Thank you, Lord, that even though my dreams crumbled, you are able to raise new dreams out of the ashes, restoring joy, hope, and purpose for my life.

Chapter 10

Gifts

The greatest gifts can be missed in the blink of an eye. They are not always obvious: time shared, compassion, and sometimes a gift cradled in another's arms.

I was the grateful recipient of such gifts. The windowsill of my sterile hospital room held ivy, flowering plants, and floral bouquets that shimmered in the sun's rays. My mom and sisters walked the halls during my surgery and waited with me for the final diagnosis.

After I returned home, two of my brothers drove up for an overnight visit. My friend Spanky flew in to spend a few days with me so my mom could go home, knowing I would not be alone.

Cards and notes encouraged me with God's grace and healing not only after surgery but also throughout the course of my chemotherapy. Gift books, devotionals, and journals lay scattered within arm's reach around my rocking chair. Soft hats and snuggly blankets enfolded me in a mantle of God's love.

We have been told laughter is the best medicine. Even though cancer is not a laughing matter, funny cards and cartoons tickled me. Raggedy Ann cheered me up after surgery. Merriment from my sister's buoyant attitude that "hats can be fun," kept me afloat as I faced chemotherapy-induced baldness.

During my tests, family and friends distracted me from escalating fears. They stayed with me in the hospital, held my hand when I cried, commiserated with me, prayed for me, and laughed with me. They delivered hot meals, took me grocery shopping, and helped with simple housekeeping chores.

Between their busy work and personal schedules, they chauffeured me to and from chemotherapy. I wasn't allowed to drive myself because of the sedative effects of my treatment. Even though they could have dropped me off, they sat by my side, books and magazines in hand, and endured the four-hour treatments while I dozed. Spanky had packed a chemo bag for me: a knit throw, jacket, book, slipper socks, and jewelry. Their love penetrated the isolation of my chemotherapy cubicle.

The people God has placed in our lives are our greatest treasures. The outpouring of love I received flowed from relationships established through the years. Encouragement, aid, and compassion—the earmarks of true friendship—were God's gifts to me.

> Dear friends, since God loved us that much, we surely ought to
> love each other. (1 John 4:11 NLT)

Prayer: Thank you, Lord, for my family and friends who stick with me through the difficult seasons, cheering me up with their presence, gifts, and laughter.

Chapter 11

BLONDE, BRUNETTE, OR RED?

I paced back and forth by the window, peering out between the curtains once again. Two weeks had passed since my cancer surgery, and my friend Spanky planned to stay with me for a few days. Housebound, I anticipated being sprung and welcomed the distraction of our way-too-fun shopping sprees.

But first, we had a more serious task at hand. I had scheduled an appointment with the American Cancer Society to be fitted with a wig. Chemotherapy loomed ahead. With Spanky's flair for fashion, I felt assured I would depart with the most flattering of styles.

Upon arrival to my appointment, an older woman welcomed us. We trailed her down a dark hallway, her clicking heels echoing down the length of the corridor. She halted before a dark wooden door and heaved it open. I peeked into the narrow office. Old wooden dressers marred with scratches lined the perimeter of the dimly lit room.

She directed me to take a seat on a vanity stool positioned in front of an antique mirror encircled with fluorescent lights. Wigs draped their respective stands: blonde, brunette, auburn, gray.

She yanked open the sticking drawers, rummaged through the contents, and pulled out brunette wigs in short and medium lengths. She balanced the wig next to my head to compare hair color. Next, she reached into a slotted box and plucked out a nylon stockinet. She gently but firmly tugged the covering over my head and stuffed my hair under the nylon band. As I gazed into the mirror, I drew in a sharp breath. A hairless reflection stared back at me.

She extracted a short bob wig from a Ziploc bag, shook it out, and fitted the hair piece over my head, combing through the synthetic fibers with her fingers. She passed me a handheld mirror and slowly rotated the stool as I appraised the selection. We repeated this process several times until we agreed upon a stylish cut. As she packaged the wig, she instructed me on its care. Her last warning—avoid steam, lest the synthetic fibers melt and clump together.

I heaved a sigh of relief. Mission accomplished. For fun, I donned wigs in various styles and colors, taking advantage of this opportunity. I modeled red curls, blonde waves, and raven-black tresses. We howled with laughter.

I clutched my new hair, thanked my benefactor, and departed. I discovered a spring in my step and a new confidence. What I'd perceived as a difficult task transformed into a fun-filled adventure. I realized I wasn't alone in this uncharted course. God had provided for me. He even interspersed laughter and joy along the way through friends and kind strangers.

> He will once again fill your mouth with laughter and your lips
> with shouts of joy. (Job 8:21 NLT)

Prayer: Thank you, Lord, for providing fun, laughter, and friends in the face of cancer. Help me to remember that you provide for me.

Chapter 12

BAG OF PROMISES

I gazed around the parking lot. A statuesque woman stepped out of her nearby sedan, crunching the orange and red leaves as they swirled to the ground beneath her feet. A black turban peeked out from underneath her black brimmed hat. She clutched her black wool jacket around her neck and strode toward the building. Was she attending my "Look Good Feel Better" class?

I poked my head around the door, slipped into the room, and took a seat at the table next to the black-clad lady. I glanced around, taking note of my fellow classmates donned in wigs and floppy crocheted hats. At each place setting, a mirror stood next to a red cosmetic satchel inscribed with "Look Good Feel Better"—a promise I desperately hoped was true. Cancer surgery had assaulted my femininity. Hair loss threatened my identity.

Tossing her shiny chestnut hair over her shoulder, our instructor introduced herself and the program. "The 'Look Good Feel Better' program is designed to build confidence in women undergoing chemotherapy through the use of makeup techniques, wigs, and head coverings."

Although she hadn't struggled with cancer, the battle had become personal when a close relative had undergone chemotherapy. Skilled in cosmetology, she undertook the mission of helping other women cope with the ravages of this disease.

Our bag of promises contained complimentary name-brand cosmetics including Lancôme, Estée Lauder, and Clinique—donated specifically for this program. As we rummaged through our bags, we extracted eye shadows, pencils, brushes, powder, base, mascara, and lipstick.

We cleansed, toned, and moisturized our faces. For the dark circles under our eyes due to chemotherapy, we used concealer. We applied foundation to smooth the imperfections in our complexions and camouflage sallow undertones. Broad strokes of blush contoured our cheekbones, giving rise to a natural warmth and glow. Lipsticks in luscious shades of pinks and wines filled in the fullness created by lip liner.

I was prepared for hair loss, but it never occurred to me that I would also lose my eyebrows and eyelashes. Our instructor demonstrated eyeliner techniques that created the illusion of lashes. By aligning the arch of the brow with the pupil of the eye, we fashioned eyebrows with our eyebrow pencils.

We laughed, chatted, swapped colors, and admired one another's results.

Amidst words of encouragement, we fitted wigs, modeled head coverings, and demonstrated scarf-tying techniques. With our red satchels in hand, we departed, empowered with promises to help us cope with the challenges that lay ahead.

Far greater than our red bag of promises are the unfailing promises of God. He will never leave us or forsake us. We are still his beautiful women.

> God's way is perfect. All the Lord's promises prove true.
> (2 Samuel 22:31 NLT)

Prayer: Thank you, Lord, that when we feel our beauty has been robbed by chemotherapy and cancer, you provide beauty treatments for your daughters. You remind us that we are still beautiful in your eyes.

Chapter 13

Fun?

"We have to make this fun!" my sister, Jean, said with a gleam in her eye.

I glared at her from my hospital bed. Fun? I hit the pain button again in hopes of deleting my abdominal pain as well as this conversation. What happened to sisterly compassion and commiseration? The doctor had just disappeared around the door, leaving me with a mishmash of information on ovarian cancer to sift through. I would rather shred and trash the literature along with the cancer.

Hats, wigs, scarves? Fun? While my niece excitedly surfed the Web for wigs, I searched for hats. But I had a problem. Most hats spun around on my petite head like a top. I stared at the heads of mannequins draped with silky swaths of chicly tied fabric. On my head, these elegant scarves slipped over my eyes and morphed into a pirate patch.

Several weeks later, I eyed the hat trees in the discount store with misgivings. Gingerly, I flicked a turquoise newsboy cap, embellished with sequins, from its perch. Standing in front of the mirror, I slipped my hair under the cap. The sequins glimmered beneath the fluorescent lights. I smiled. I had found the perfect hat. As I plucked one hat after another from its roost, I beamed at my reflection in the mirror. Red hats, blue hats, wool hats, cloche hats.

I plopped hats over wigs, tugged hats over turbans, and pulled hats over my bald head. Before long, I crammed a duffel bag with hats. At Christmas, my sisters, in-laws, and nieces rifled through my bag. Giggling, each one stuffed her hair under the brim of a hat and modeled her new fashion statement for a group picture.

My sister was right. Hats and wigs were fun.

I will turn their mourning into gladness. (Jeremiah 31:13 NIV)

Prayer: Thank you, Lord, for providing fun in the midst of my crisis. Please help me to maintain a sense of humor and the ability to laugh despite the gravity of cancer.

Chapter 14

Helpful Hints: Chemo Day

1. Wear comfy, loose clothes and dress in layers for temperature variations.

2. Clothing should allow easy access to your arms for IV placement or your port.

3. Take a favorite throw or pillow for comfort.

4. Bring slippers or warm socks.

5. Eat a light meal before your treatment.

6. Pack light snacks or favorite beverages. Juices, soda, and crackers may be provided. Check with your clinic.

7. Some treatments take several hours, so bring along books, magazines, computer, DVDs, or an iPad.

8. Arrange a ride for your first treatment, and every treatment, if driving is contraindicated with your chemotherapy protocol.

9. Alert the staff if you experience any new or unusual symptoms.

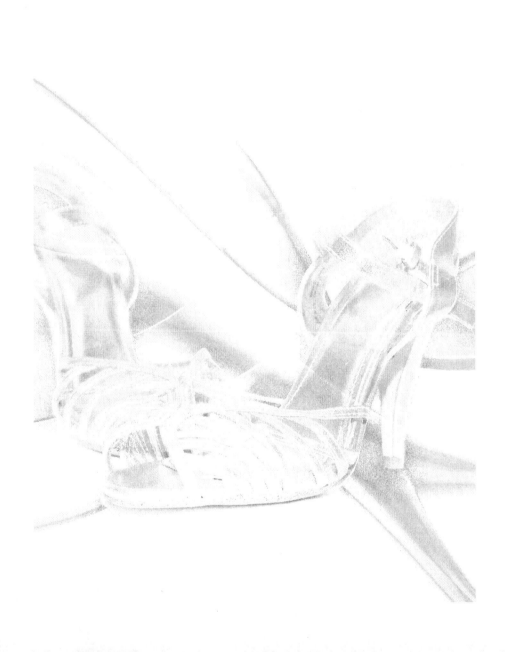

Chapter 15

WHERE ARE YOU, GOD?

A drizzly overcast sky greeted me as I steeled myself for the first of six chemotherapy treatments. I glanced around my living room, searching for any stray items I'd forgotten to pack. My friend Spanky had presented me with a purple bag filled with the basics for chemotherapy comfort: a blue and green afghan, a fancy sweatshirt, lavender slipper socks, and two devotional books. Amethyst earrings and a coin pearl necklace added bling to bolster my confidence.

While waiting for Kathy, I pressed my face against the cold windowpane. Worry from the possible side effects of chemotherapy dominated my thoughts. I'd heard all about the nausea, vomiting, fatigue, body aches, and a life-threatening allergic reaction. My nerves felt jangled. Sleep had eluded me. *Maybe this won't be so bad. Some people breeze through their chemotherapy.*

As the nurse led me to a curvy lounge chair, soft laughter and chatter drifted from a nearby cubicle. She tucked me in with pillows and blankets. To pop up a vein for IV placement, she wrapped a heating pad around my arm. I extended my hands to receive the needle that would carry these cancer-destroying drugs into my body. A poison that would indiscriminately destroy healthy tissue as well as the cancer.

My nurse poised a pediatric needle over my narrow veins. At the poke, I grimaced. A picture of Jesus's nail-pierced hands flashed through my mind. Like a toxic poison, he had taken upon himself the sin of the world. I considered how tiny my needle and how minute the skin prick was when compared to the hands of our Savior, impaled with rusty nails.

The IV pump clicked. Pre-meds to avert nausea and an allergic reaction dripped into my vein. The nurse hung my chemotherapy bag, keeping a watchful eye on me and the machines I was hooked up to.

A few moments later, my heart raced. My chest pounded. The nurse stopped the chemotherapy. My doctor and several nurses rushed in and surrounded my chair. The doctor ordered stronger medication to stave off further side effects. Under even closer surveillance, they resumed my chemotherapy. They also extended my infusion time from four to six hours.

I groaned.

While the chemotherapy dripped into my veins, I dozed. Kathy prayed. As the treatment progressed, my legs grew restless. I hauled my woozy body out of the chair. Leaning on my IV pole for support, I trudged around the periphery of the unit. But I found no relief as I fidgeted and shifted between chairs. Finally, the medication had infused, and Kathy drove me home. I crawled into bed and allowed the lingering sedation to lull me to sleep.

The next day, my head spun, and my stomach churned with the slightest movement. Two days later, my joints ached. Nothing prepared me for the agony of shooting nerve and crushing chest pain. With every movement, every breath, the intensity increased. I downed the painkillers with little relief. *I don't think I can go through this again. Where are you, God?*

My muscles quivered like gelatin. Gelatin. It sounded, oh, so good, but fatigue overwhelmed me before the water boiled. Profound muscle weakness limited my sitting to ten-minute intervals. I dragged myself between the bed and the couch. A fog had settled over my mind. I couldn't read. I couldn't pray. I couldn't even focus on television or my favorite movies. All I could do was rest and trust God with childlike faith.

> Have mercy on me, my God, have mercy on me, for in you I take refuge. I will take refuge in the shadow of your wings until the disaster has passed. (Psalm 57:1 NIV)

Prayer: O Lord, I'm so frightened. Please hold back the torrents of fear that threaten to overwhelm me. Help me to survive the side effects of my treatment.

Chapter 16

Helpful Hints: Hair Loss

1. Select a wig before you lose your hair, in order to match your color and style. Clip a lock of hair for future purchases.

2. If your hair is long, you may want to trim it short to reduce the amount of hair shed.

3. Shave or not to shave? It's a personal preference of how to deal with the barren patches and the wisps. Shaving will help if hair loss is physically painful.

4. Hair loss involves all areas of body hair including eyelashes, eyebrows, and pubic hair.

5. Enroll in the "Look Good Feel Better" program offered through the American Cancer Society. The class covers makeup tips, including the illusion of eyebrows and lashes, scarf-tying techniques, and wigs. They also provide you with a bag of free name-brand makeup and facial products.

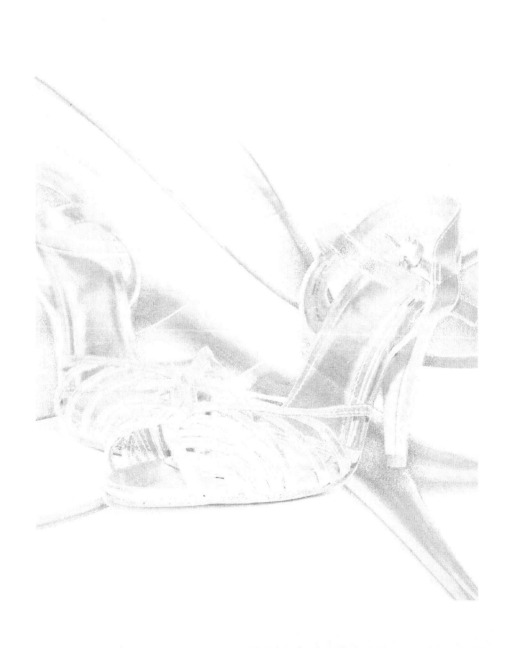

Chapter 17

BALD IS BEAUTIFUL

"It's time," I said to my friend, Kathy.

Chest aching, I choked back the sobs. As I gazed at my reflection in the mirror, hot tears rolled down my cheeks, splashing the vanity. Barren patches of scalp had replaced my fine brown hair.

Over the course of several days, hair clumped and clogged the shower drain. Strands of it clung to my pillow and glistened in the sunlight, mocking me. Hair tangled and matted the teeth of my comb. When I shampooed, hundreds of needle pricks shot through my scalp. As the rustling breezes tousled my hair, I winced in pain. No one had told me that hair loss could be so physically painful.

The previous month, I had told my hairdresser I had cancer. With a deep sigh, she firmly rested her hands on my shoulders. She bent her head down next to mine and gazed into my eyes through the mirror.

Her voice wavered, "I have styled your hair for over twenty-five years. It's my place to shave your head when you are ready."

She gripped my shoulders and pressed her cheek next to mine. I nodded. With the back of her hand, she brushed away the tears pooling in her eyes.

The time had arrived to shave my head. Silence permeated the vehicle as Kathy drove me to the salon. My hairdresser greeted me with a hug and guided us to a private corner. The fruity odor of all the hair products I wouldn't need wafted by my nostrils. I hung my head.

The buzz of the razor resonated in my ears. I squeezed my eyes shut, but tears escaped anyway, splattering my cape. With one hand, I clutched Kathy's. I gripped the armrest with the other.

"Joanie, you need to look," Kathy whispered.

I forced my eyes open and peeked at my reflection in the mirror. As the brush of the blades sliced what little hair I had left, sharp pain radiated through my scalp. I blinked back more tears. The last wisps of hair dropped onto my cape, floated to the floor and scattered around my chair, only to be swept away and trashed. Was God counting each hair as it fell? I hoped so.

Through misty eyes, I stared at the bald woman in the mirror, only to discover that she was me.

"Bald is beautiful," the young woman on the television screen stated as she proudly displayed her bald head.

She too had ovarian cancer followed by chemotherapy. Television stations aired this commercial during the entire course of my treatment. I wasn't alone. I held on to this message like a child clutching a favorite teddy bear. Words of comfort and hope wrapped themselves around me. I allowed God's peace to settle over me and grabbed hold of a new-found courage. *I can do this.*

Yes, bald is beautiful. But even more importantly, I was still beautiful in God's eyes.

> To all who mourn in Israel he will give a crown of beauty for ashes, a joyous blessing instead of mourning, festive praise instead of despair. (Isaiah 61:3 NLT)

Prayer: Lord, I thank you for my friends who hold my hand and walk with me through the hard places. Please give me the strength and courage I need to face the days ahead.

Chapter 18

Two Paths

"I don't think I can do this again," I told my doctor as I slumped over in the chair. I had completed my first course of chemotherapy, pummeled by pain, fatigue, and nausea. Now I faced a second round.

With his warm, brown eyes, he studied my face, leaned toward me, and cupped his burly hand over mine. "You can stop any time."

I drew back. Stunned. Confused. Chemotherapy—a choice? End the gnawing pain, debilitating weakness, and nausea? Two paths loomed before me. Each presented its bitter cup, but from one I must drink. The original course offered a bittersweet poison, a chemotherapy cocktail. But a second path emerged—no treatment. A path on which I feared recurrence. If left unchecked, the cancer could spread like an acrid nightshade vine that invades and chokes out the surrounding vegetation. In this case—my life.

In my mind's eye, I strained to see my future, but the outlook remained obscure. I don't like ambiguity. I wanted an accurate forecast, only I wasn't dealing with the weather but with my life.

I felt blindfolded like Lady Justice. The balancing scales weighed the pros and cons. I remembered the Lord's words to me, "Go through the process." The scales tipped. Yes, for me chemotherapy was the right path if I wanted to live. I needed to know I'd done everything possible to kill the cancer, and to not be haunted later by "what ifs."

I straightened my spine, pulled my shoulders back, and drew in a deep breath. Armed with fresh courage, I grabbed my purple satchel and strode into the treatment room. Once again, the nurse inserted the needle and infused the chemotherapy into my vein. I dug in my heels and clenched my teeth, steeling myself for the onslaught of pain and fatigue that would once again ensue.

Even though I was uncertain of where this path would lead, I knew God would walk with me and guide me. Courage didn't mean I wasn't afraid, but I pressed forward despite the fear. I reminded myself of the words inscribed on a plaque, "God will never lead you where his grace cannot keep you."

Chemotherapy was the path God chose for me. In my frailty, I cried out for his strength and grace as I continued my course.

> He guides me along the right paths for his name's sake. (Psalm 23:3 NIV)

Prayer: Lord, help me to trust you when I'm afraid and don't know which path to choose. Be my guide and keep me on your path.

Chapter 19

A Chemo Christmas

My Christmas preparations had sputtered to a grinding halt. Chemotherapy interrupted my scurrying on the never-ending treadmill of holiday festivities. Instead of a Christmas letter brimming with the clever antics of children and pets, I announced that I had cancer.

I decorated sparsely that year. A simple hand-painted nativity set graced my fireplace mantel. Multi-colored lights surrounded the figurines, casting shadows along the pale wall. As I faced another round of chemotherapy, the Christmas lights mounted a valiant attempt to cheer me. Cancer surgery had prevented me from traveling for Thanksgiving, so I was looking forward to going home for Christmas.

My mom and sister drove up and stayed with me during my chemotherapy treatment the week before Christmas. The next day, under overcast skies, we traveled the four hours home. The flat farmlands, dotted with straw stubble, reflected the dormancy of my life.

On Christmas Eve, the joyous strains of Christmas carols echoed through the vaulted church ceiling—the glory of Christmas. In the candlelight, rainbows reflected and danced in the facets of my crystal jewelry. Truly a light had shone in the darkness.

The next week, the rest of my family descended upon us.

I rocked in the recliner with my niece's fluffy white froufrou dog on my lap. She'd been groomed, clipped, and had a bow perched between her ears.

With the arrival of each new family, including two more dogs, the decibels rose. The match was on with yipping, barking, and growling until relegated to their respective corners.

After dinner, we drew numbers and tore into the white elephant gifts. Amidst gaiety and laughter, we shook, selected, stole, and re-stole packages until all were claimed.

My family modeled my hats—paraded, posed, and photographed. Late night chats, games, and fanfare abruptly ended as each family departed. Soon, I also would head back home to face another round of chemotherapy.

Despite a Christmas of grappling with the unfamiliar world of cancer and chemotherapy, one thing hadn't changed. God is the same yesterday, today and forever. He sent his Son, a baby born in a manger on Christmas morning. Emmanuel—God with us. And he was still with me.

> Jesus Christ is the same yesterday and today and forever. (Hebrews 13:8 NIV)

Prayer: Even though I am unable to celebrate Christmas in my usual fashion, I thank you, Lord, that the truth of the Christmas message never changes—a Savior was born, Christ the Lord.

Chapter 20

A Thief in the Night

Pain—stalked me by day and pounced at night.

Throbbed. Ached. Stabbed.

Pain—a fire-breathing serpent that gnawed at me with its teeth and stung with its tail. An unrelenting torment that could drive even the sanest to the brink of insanity.

No medication, massage, or outpouring of tears provided relief. Just as my bald head sank into the pillow, my nerves fired waves of throbbing pain throughout my toe. The appendage felt inflamed and inflated like a red, swollen balloon ready to pop. I scrunched my stomach muscles and rocked back and forth, rumpling the sheets. Pain crushed my chest. *Am I having a heart attack?* No, the doctor had said that the chest pain resulted from chemotherapy-induced demolition of my bone marrow. Besides, the stabbing had eased since the last dose of my pain medication. Sleep eluded me.

Pain—a thief in the night.

Exhausted, I faded into a twilight sleep. Beneath my aching sternum, my heart hammered. My eyes flew open. Steam billowed from my scalp as if I had been thrust into a sauna. Sweat beaded on my brow and dripped down my flushed cheeks. As my trembling hand groped for the fan, I tossed the blankets to the floor in a crumpled heap.

Hormones had seized my body as if declaring in alien voices, "Resistance is futile."

Soon, clammy chills replaced the flashes of heat. Shivering, I tugged the blankets around my shoulders. All too soon, the cycle began again.

Hot flashes—a thief in the night.

My nerve impulses heightened as if multi-legged creatures raced beneath my skin. Worst-case scenarios wrapped around my mind, clinging with their octopus tentacles.

I wrestled to break the suction of one fear only to find another had latched on. With a gnarly finger, unsolicited questions beckoned me. *What will my future hold? Will I survive? What if …?* Worry, doubt, and fear—the runaway trains that transport their passengers on an unbidden ride.

Anxiety—a thief in the night.

I draped my arm over my head. The slightest movement provoked waves of nausea. Like a roller coaster climbing the track, clackety-clacking toward the inevitable plunge, my stomach churned and lurched. I lunged for the cold porcelain, poised mockingly like a throne.

Nausea—a thief in the night.

Chemotherapy robbed me of sleep, deprived me of comfort, and tormented me with pain, fear, and doubts. I questioned God. *Why don't you stop the pain? Why must I suffer like this?*

But God helped me cope. He reminded me to take my pain and nausea medications around the clock. When I told my doctor about critters crawling beneath my skin, he prescribed anti-anxiety medication, which helped to restore my sanity and calm my fears.

I discovered I wasn't alone. God was with me even if he didn't answer my prayers the way I wanted him to. Between the blasts of chemotherapy, he provided me oases of rest. I felt his peace as I rested during the day, curled up on the couch. I sensed arms wrapped around me as he comforted me and cradled me like a small child. His child.

In the meantime, I snatched whatever sleep I could as I shuffled between my bed, couch, and chair. *Maybe tonight will be better,* I'd hope. But I knew that whatever my night would bring, God would be with me and help me to cope.

> Praise be to the God and Father of our Lord Jesus Christ, the Father of compassion and the God of all comfort, who comforts us in all our troubles, so that we can comfort those in any trouble with the comfort we ourselves receive from God. (2 Corinthians 1:3-4 NIV)

Prayer: Lord, even when I don't feel your presence, I know you're always near. You never abandon me or forsake me. Thank you, Lord, for giving me strategies to cope with the side effects of chemotherapy.

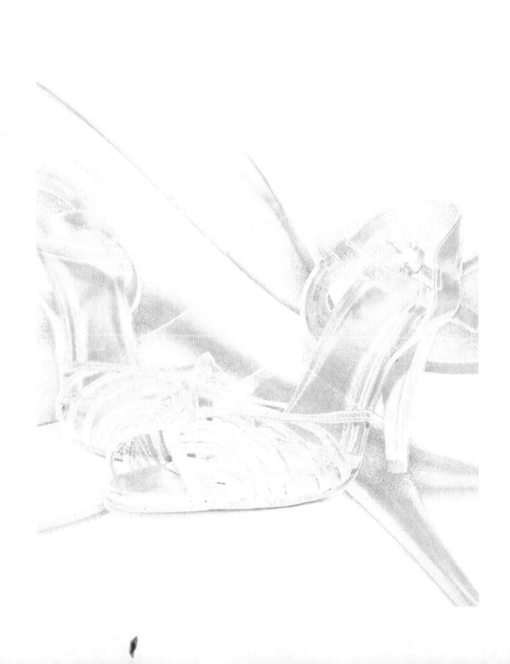

Chapter 21

HOME!

I clutched my chest. My knees buckled. I slumped over and leaned against a cold rock wall. I had made a terrible mistake.

Ten days had passed since my fourth round of chemotherapy. Claustrophobic and stir-crazy, I finally felt strong enough to go for a walk. I had pulled on my purple jacket and yanked a knit cap over my bald head. With its deceptive warmth, the brightness of the winter sun lured me outdoors. The crisp air stung my nostrils. Gusts of wind whipped around me and stirred the barren branches. Shivering, I picked up my pace.

About a half-mile out, pain gripped my sternum. I gasped. Between staggered breaths, I scanned down the street searching for a bench on which to rest. Frantically, I thrust my hand into my pockets—no cell phone, no money. *How am I going to get home?* I gazed longingly at the buses that rumbled past, belching black smoke laced with diesel fumes.

Panting, I coaxed my wobbly legs to cross the street. *Just put one foot in front of the other.* Weak and dizzy, I crumpled onto a cold, metal bus bench and dropped my throbbing head between my knees. My heart pounded. My muscles quivered, each fiber stretched like strings on a musical instrument.

I waited for the heaviness in my chest to lift and then continued my trek. Another block. Another bench. Two blocks to go.

My hands trembled as I jabbed the key into the lock. I let my hat and coat slip to the floor and flopped onto the couch, breathless and exhausted. As my breathing eased, I thanked God that he had brought me safely home.

During the remainder of my treatments, I didn't venture out on foot. I hadn't realized how much the cumulative effects of chemotherapy had taken a toll on my stamina. I'm grateful God guided me home even when I unknowingly pushed my limits.

Strengthen the feeble hands, steady the knees that give way; say to those with fearful hearts, "Be strong, do not fear; your God will come." (Isaiah 35:3-4 NIV)

Prayer: Thank you, Lord, for strengthening me when I am weak.

Chapter 22

WHERE, O WHERE HAS MY ENERGY GONE?

I dragged the vacuum out of the closet and stood it in the hallway. Winded, I stumbled to my rocker. I turned and glared at my nemesis. Who would have thought that pushing my lightweight sweeper could consume so much energy and strength? Friends stopped by and vacuumed while I looked on, slumped over in a nearby chair. Even light housekeeping tasks—mopping, laundry, and cooking—demanded frequent stopovers in my rocker and concluded with a nap. The duster lay neglected on the shelf, a constant reminder of my new collector's item—dust bunnies.

In the grocery store, I draped my arms over the cart and lumbered down the aisles. With no warning, dizziness and fatigue descended upon me. My leg muscles quivered. I teetered and grabbed hold of the handles on the cart. Despite the remaining items on my list, I staggered to the checkout. *I have to leave now!*

Back home, I dropped the bags in the hallway and stumbled to the couch. Hopefully, my frozen food remained nestled in a no-thaw zone until I could drag the groceries to the freezer.

My ladies' Bible study was scheduled the next day. Shower, makeup, wig. I was all dressed but too worn out to go. Like a ruthless flu virus, exhaustion struck again. My chest throbbed. I kicked off my shoes and flopped onto the bed, hoping my clothes wouldn't wrinkle. *Maybe if I rested … just a bit, I could still go …* I had promised to bring bagels, so I hauled myself out of bed, slipped into my shoes and coat and grabbed my keys.

At the bagel shop, the person ahead of me stood for what seemed like forever at the counter. *Hurry up!* My head spun. I scanned the shop, searching for a solid surface to hold me upright. No counter to grasp, no free wall to lean against. My legs trembled. Finally, the clerk took my order.

Clutching my bagels and cream cheese, I stumbled to the car and stuck the key into the lock. The latch wouldn't budge. I glanced inside the vehicle. *This isn't my car!* Peeking over my shoulder I scanned the lot. No one in sight. My car, the same color and style, sat two spaces over in the parking lot.

I trudged over to my vehicle, clicked the key in the lock, slid behind the wheel, and arrived at my Bible study with bagels and wild berry cream cheese.

Each subsequent chemotherapy treatment siphoned my strength. I never fully recharged between treatments. The barrage of debilitating weakness thwarted my plans and frustrated me. *Will I ever feel better?*

I knew that the exhaustion was temporary, but throughout chemotherapy, fatigue remained my daily reality. *Rest*. This was the Lord's word for me. *Rest*. So, I reluctantly laid aside my to-do list and learned to be still and to rest in him.

Come to me, all you who are weary and burdened, and I will give you rest. (Matthew 11:28 NIV)

Prayer: Lord, I feel so frustrated when I can't do the things I've always done with ease. Now, even the simplest tasks seem overwhelming. Thank you for providing help and offering me your rest during this season.

Chapter 23

Uncovered!

My next hurdle? Would I allow anyone to see me bald? On one hand, I didn't care, but would the discomfort of others cause me to feel uncomfortable? Could I bear their turning away, shocked and embarrassed? Before they averted their eyes, would I catch a glimpse of pity? I made my decision. I vowed to keep my head covered.

Once I adjusted to the no-hair look, I enjoyed mixing and matching hats, wigs, and turbans. I changed the color and length of my hair by slipping hair accents under my hat brims. "Hair" care proved simple. I dabbed shampoo on my head and massaged a drop of conditioner into my scalp to moisturize the bare skin.

In the middle of my chemotherapy, three of my college friends and I scheduled our annual reunion, celebrating thirty years since graduation. I drove two hours to meet my friends at a lake house in the Galena territories. Our rental home cozied up to woodlands, home to red-crested woodpeckers, gray squirrels, and white-tailed deer. In the quaint town nearby, we dodged a cold drizzle as we shopped the boutiques and specialty stores that lined the cobblestone sidewalks.

That evening, we grilled steaks and dined by candlelight. Despite the freezing rain, we hopped into the hot tub. I had pulled a white cap trimmed with navy lace over my bald head. A mantle of steam hovered over the Jacuzzi, wafting a chemical odor that rankled my nostrils. Just beyond the woods, a small lake echoed our chatter and laughter.

After the soothing jets relaxed our tired muscles, we donned our fleece robes and fuzzy slippers. Reminiscing, we lounged around the fireplace, warmed by the crackling blaze. A chilly draft grazed my scalp. My hand automatically brushed my head. I forgot to cover my baldness! I shot a quick glance at each face that glowed in the light from the flickering flames. No shocked expressions. No one seemed to notice. I sank into the couch, sipped my tea, and allowed the warmth of our friendships to mingle with the coziness of the flames lapping the logs with glee.

I realized that with or without hair, baldness did not determine my identity. Despite the years of life's diverse trials and joys, we were all still the same people. Our friendships, cemented in the midst of dorm life, remained strong.

A friend loves at all times. (Proverbs 17:17 NIV)

Prayer: Lord, thank you for family and friends who stand with me in my trials.

Chapter 24

WHO SWITCHED OFF MY BRAIN?

Chemo brain—the impenetrable fog that settled over my mind. The haze reminded me of my trip to Mount Rainier. During our descent along the mountain's winding roads, a low cloud ceiling enshrouded us beneath an opaque film. The cascading waterfalls, lush foliage, and purple wildflowers, so vibrant when greeting us upon our arrival, now lay hidden within the cloud cover—inaccessible like my memory.

Chemotherapy had short-circuited my brain. The synaptic gaps widened like a cog in a wheel with broken and worn projections, failing to engage the next gear, grinding to a halt. Delayed and disorganized nerve conduction plagued me as I tried to complete simple tasks.

I grappled for a name on the blank slate of my mind, able to greet long-time acquaintances with nothing but a plastered-on smile. Embarrassed, I would fumble for the right words, but my tongue seemed to dangle from my gaping mouth. Mid-sentence, my train of thought vanished. *Focus. Concentrate.*

Memory lapses disrupted my mindless routines. I strode into rooms only to stop abruptly, staring because I'd forgotten why I crossed the threshold. Treasures I squirreled away for safekeeping seemed to disappear into black holes. With a diminished capacity for concentration, I reached into the recesses of my mind to grab hold of an informational nugget someone had shared with me, only to come up empty-handed. Stored knowledge from years of study and rote training remained irretrievable. The marriage between my bank statement and my balance had succumbed to irreconcilable differences. How does two plus two equal five?

I don't know who switched off my brain, but I've learned ways to cope during my recovery. Until the fog lifted and my brain circuitry reconnected, I memorized, made lists, pored over procedures until I understood, read until I comprehended, and practiced until I accomplished. I double checked the locks on doors, the controls on my stove, and only heated water in a tea kettle that whistled.

Despite the mental challenges, I reminded myself that I have the mind of Christ. When I asked for help with my memory, the Holy Spirit was my reminder.

But we have the mind of Christ. (1 Corinthians 2:16 NIV)

Prayer: Thank you, Lord, that when my thinking processes seem clouded, you help clarify my thoughts and remind me of all I need to know. Please help me to be patient with myself when my mind seems slow and forgetful.

Chapter 25

TAKEN BY SURPRISE

A towering basket of lavender nearly hid my manager's grin as she stood in the doorway of my home several weeks after my surgery. I slipped back the lavender cellophane, revealing lavender towels, lavender sachets, a soft white blanket, and a microwaveable heating wrap. The generosity of my co-workers overwhelmed me, as did my manager who took time out of her busy schedule to personally deliver this lovely gift.

My supervisor settled in a chair while I set the basket on a nearby table. We discussed the course of my surgery and the upcoming chemotherapy. I felt her support and encouragement—until she stated, "According to policy, we are unable to hold your position. You will be temporarily displaced."

My stomach recoiled as if punched with a fist.

"Nothing personal," she reassured me. "Just a formality."

Not personal? I've essentially lost my job!

"We'll send you a certified letter regarding your temporary displacement," she continued. "When you're ready to return to work, we'll make every effort to locate a comparable position."

Already burdened with the fears and doubts of cancer and chemotherapy, I added a new worry—a job. I tried to live one day at a time, but anxiety threatened to suck me into its murky pool. Even though I wasn't ready to return to work, my future employment hovered over me like storm clouds gathering on the horizon.

Over the next few months, I wrestled with fear, anger, resentment, and worry. I reminded myself that God did not give me the grace today to deal with tomorrow. I prayed for the right position to open. I needed to fellowship with God, not with my problem.

Despite the lingering weakness and fatigue, I sensed the time had come to check the job postings. Six months had passed since my surgery and one month since I completed my last chemotherapy treatment. I drove to the Human Resources office and scrolled down the computerized list. *I don't believe it!* The job I had sought before my diagnosis was listed in the seven-day postings. Therefore, my seniority would be considered in the transfer. A few days either way, I would have missed this opportunity.

I applied for the position and got the job. God was faithful. His timing was perfect.

> For great is his love toward us, and the faithfulness of the Lord endures forever. Praise the Lord. (Psalm 117:2 NIV)

Prayer: Lord, I thank you for the surprises you bring me at just the right time. Help me to see that nothing can stand in the way of your perfect plans and purposes for me.

Chapter 26

Dark Shadow

A mirror never lies. The reflective pane mimics a magnifying glass with a zoom lens designed to enhance every spot, wrinkle, blemish, and roll. I scrutinized my eyelashes. Stripped bare. Three nut-brown strands of hair graced each eyebrow.

A dark shadow hovered over my scalp. *What is this dirt on my head?* I had just dabbed a drop of shampoo on my bald head in the shower. I rubbed the top of my head, attempting to brush away the dirt. Soft bristles tickled my palm. I squealed. Hair!

I anticipated the promised curls, courtesy of chemotherapy. Curling irons, rollers, or perm solutions had created every ringlet that framed my face. The thought of sporting natural curls thrilled me. But there was one problem. My hair defied the odds and reappeared straight and fine. Once again, curls eluded me. Instead, my hair boasted platinum blonde frosted tips.

When I returned to work, my hair growth had progressed to stubble. Since hats were not allowed, I wore a wig. My wig shifted on my head and crept up the nape of my neck. I yanked and readjusted, only to find it askew again.

My brassy hair barely covered my scalp, but Spanky encouraged me to ditch the wigs. My hair had never been chopped this short. Despite the itching and sweating from the wig, I persisted with my synthetic hair for two more weeks.

Finally, I screwed up my courage to be seen in public with cropped hair. My hair had grown back with bleach-blonde tips and flaunted perfect summer highlights courtesy of chemotherapy.

With reluctance, I faced my co-workers. No dropped jaws. No embarrassing stares. Instead, I received countless compliments on my frosted hair with requests for the name of my hairdresser.

Freed from wigs and hats, I welcomed the cool evening breezes that ruffled my closely trimmed hair. No scalp pain! Soon my eyebrows returned with no plucking required. My eyelashes reappeared, though too stubby and sparse to be featured in a mascara commercial.

Like crocus buds that burst forth from the once frozen ground and herald the arrival of spring, the regeneration of my hair signaled the restoration of my health.

You restored me to health and let me live. (Isaiah 38:16 NIV)

Prayer: Thank you, Lord, for renewed hope arising from the appearance of new hair, a sign that my winter is over, and spring has arrived.

Chapter 27

THE RACE

The pounding of my heart reverberated in my ears. I glanced behind, but my vision clouded as beads of sweat dripped into my eyes. My feet beat the pavement while my opponent, cancer, clipped my heels. His steamy breath blasted my neck. My chest heaved, and my stomach cramped. I crossed the finish line. I won the race. My follow-up tests for ovarian cancer were negative.

The race against cancer got underway before each follow-up appointment. The tension mounted throughout each nerve fiber, like a stretched rubber band. Beneath my calm façade, the assault of fear and anxiety rumbled. The thunder of "what if?" resonated through my mind and pummeled my faith.

Friends prayed for me. Once again, my focus turned toward God. His peace flowed through my jangled nerves. My faith and trust were restored. As the muscle fibers relaxed, the knots dissolved in my shoulders and neck. I believed God had delivered me from cancer. I took a deep breath. I was ready to face my follow-up exam.

Once again, my feet struck the pavement. I have maintained a comfortable lead in my race against cancer with a steady stride. The clamor of my opponent has faded. The winds of adversity that once roared in my ears have transformed into a gentle breeze. With each subsequent doctor's appointment, the tension eased.

"I'm here for my social visit," I announced to my doctor.

He returned my smile as he replied, "Let's keep it that way."

> Peace I leave with you; my peace I give you. I do not give to you as the world gives. Do not let your hearts be troubled and do not be afraid. (John 14:27 NIV)

Prayer: Lord, follow-up appointments are scary. Thank you for calming my anxious heart and surrounding me with your peace. When I am afraid, help me to trust in you.

Chapter 28

HOPE DEFERRED

Thanksgiving heralded the arrival of stuffed turkey, stuffed shopping bags, and my stuffed luggage nearly packed for the drive home. I had much to be thankful for—five years without a trace of ovarian cancer. My yearly mammogram results remained pending, but I was unconcerned. While juggling shoes and socks, the phone interrupted my packing. I dived for the handset, shoes tumbling out of my arms.

A pleasant voice on the other end said, "The radiologist would like to schedule another mammogram with additional views and an ultrasound."

I froze. "What do you mean—more tests?" My dry mouth stumbled over the words. "What did he find?"

Unable to provide further information, she referred me to my doctor.

My stomach knotted. I took deep breaths to calm myself. I knew ovarian cancer increased my risk for breast cancer. With trembling hands, I punched in my doctor's phone number and paced the floor while the receptionist referred me to the nurse.

"Let me scroll through your radiology report," she said. "The radiologist noted a new density in one view. I don't think there's anything to be alarmed about," she reassured me. "Usually, the additional views are negative for malignancy. This happens to me each time."

As I hung up the phone, the Lord's quieting presence rested upon me. I drew in a deep breath. No matter the results, I would be okay.

With my five-year survival celebration on hold, I drove home for Thanksgiving. I refused to allow the holiday to be ruined by a bad report.

IN HER SHOES: DANCING IN THE SHADOW OF CANCER

Back in town for my repeat mammogram, I knew the drill—the cold, smashing machine, hold my breath by volition or by pain, a mechanical whir, release, breathe, repeat. The technician escorted me to a sitting room enveloped in a calming sea-blue décor. Wrapped in a thin, printed gown, I perched on the edge of a loveseat facing two blue wing-backed chairs. I waited for the ultrasound, frequently glancing at the clock.

The technician returned. "The radiologist is satisfied with the images. You don't need an ultrasound," she said. "You're free to go."

Waves of relief and gratitude washed over me as I sank into the depths of the blue flowered cushions.

Now I could celebrate the cure.

> You have done many good things for me, Lord, just as you promised. (Psalm 119:65 NLT)

Prayer: Lord, I am so easily frightened by bad reports. Thank you for your faithfulness and calming peace amidst the turmoil.

Part 2

Cathie: Non-Hodgkin's Lymphoma

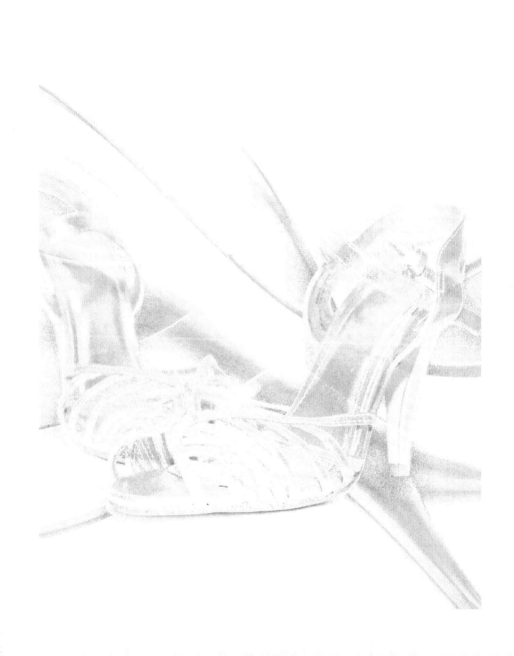

Chapter 29

THIS IS NOT NORMAL!

Cathie massaged the ache in her left arm as she walked at a brisk pace down the country road bordered by farmland. *It's just stress,* she reassured herself. Her husband had recently left his partnership and started a new business.

A chilly spring wind swept over the barren fields. Cathie shivered. She tugged her jacket a little tighter, but the warmth of the jacket was no match for the coolness that had crept into her marriage. Her struggles at home had taken a toll.

Spring gave way to a busy summer. She accepted a new position as school principal. Between her job transition, baseball, and her three boys preparing pigs and cows to show at the 4-H fair, she managed to squeeze in time one Wednesday evening to stain the basement floor of their ranch home.

After she finished, she noticed her left arm was swollen twice the size of her right arm. Even though the limb was puffy, she had no pain.

She phoned her regular doctor, an OB/GYN, and told him about the swelling. He was leaving for the day and sent her to the emergency room.

The ER physician said, "Ma'am, you're perfectly healthy. You're in great shape."

"That's the problem," Cathie said. "My arm isn't normally this size." She extended her arm toward him.

The doctor took hold of her wrist and examined her arm. He reached for her other arm and compared their circumferences. "Your one arm is definitely larger than the other. We need to schedule you for a doppler ultrasound."

"Let's do it Monday," Cathie said. "My week is pretty full, with the boys showing livestock at the 4-H fair and playing baseball."

By the following day, the swelling had increased.

Her husband strode into their room. "You're packing a bag," he noted.

"I'm going to the hospital. Something's not right," Cathie told him. "And I'm not coming home until I have some answers."

She sent her husband to the 4-H fair with two of their sons while she accompanied her middle son to his baseball game. After the game, she dropped off her son at her mother-in-law's and headed to the local emergency room.

Cathie checked herself in at the emergency room. The staff escorted her to a room, handed her a gown, and instructed her to lie down on the cart.

"You need to get my doctor here now," Cathie said to the emergency room staff. She didn't want to be seen by another doctor she didn't know who thought she was fine.

"What if we can't reach him?"

"I'm walking out," Cathie said.

"We can't just release you. You need to be checked out by a doctor."

Thankfully, Cathie's doctor arrived. He remained at her side until two o'clock a.m. During her stay, a technician performed a doppler ultrasound. The test indicated a tumor in her chest. The doctors surmised that the swelling in her arm was due to blood clots caused by the tumor.

Her doctor admitted her to the hospital, started her on anticoagulants, and scheduled a chest CT.

The next morning, her doctor arrived at six o'clock. "Cathie, you have cancer."

"They haven't even done a CT scan yet," Cathie said. "How do you know I have cancer?"

"The tumor in your chest is the size of a grapefruit. I guarantee you have cancer," the doctor said. "You'll go through with the CT scan, but the test will verify that the mass is cancer." He paused. "Cathie, I know it's cancer."

After the CT scan, her doctor gave her the choice of staying at the small local hospital or transferring to a larger medical center. Since her doctor, an OB/GYN, couldn't treat the cancer, she chose the regional cancer center.

She phoned her parents with the latest updates. They arrived several hours later and drove her to the medical facility near their home. Tension mounted. Cathie had lost an aunt and a cousin to cancer.

She spent five days in the hospital undergoing further tests that included a biopsy of the chest tumor. Since they were unable to obtain enough tissue the first time, they performed a second biopsy.

The samples confirmed the presence of cancer cells—non-Hodgkin's lymphoma.

> Hear my prayer, LORD; let my cry for help come to you. (Psalm 102:1 NIV)

Prayer: Thank you, Lord, for bringing the right people at the right time to help me. You heard me when I cried out to you for help.

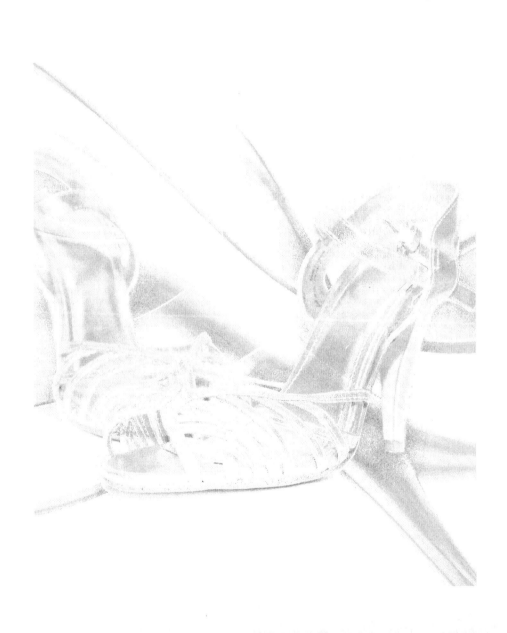

Chapter 30

THE LUNCHEON

Cathie edged her quivering body away from the kitchen sink splattered with the regurgitated remnants of her breakfast. Sucking in a deep breath, she smoothed her straight knee-length skirt and matching jacket. She stared at her reflection in the mirror and pinched her sallow cheeks. Her trembling hands glided lipstick over her pale lips. She shook the reddish-blonde wig and pulled it over her bald head, combing her fingers through the locks. *I won't miss a single day of school because of cancer.*

"Don't eat anything," she mumbled to herself. "You just have to get through this luncheon."

Cathie slipped on her pumps and grabbed her purse. As she marched out of the farmhouse, she glared at the Longaberger basket overflowing with get-well cards. Curiosity seekers from years past had swooped in, cloaked as well-wishers. The once-comforting best wishes had twisted into last wishes as the news of her lymphoma spread.

Through gritted teeth, she spat, "I will not die," and slammed the door shut.

Her first day as a middle school principal was not the day to fight chemotherapy-induced nausea. The staff planned a luncheon—a meet and greet for the entire faculty to celebrate the beginning of the school year. Conversations and activity buzzed around the room as Cathie found her seat at the table, surrounded by her new colleagues: the school superintendent and other administrators—all males.

The clamor of metal lids announced the arrival of dinner: roast beef, mashed potatoes, and gravy. The pungent odor permeated the air. Cathie's stomach lurched. She gagged and flung her hand over her mouth. *God, get me through this.*

She plastered a smile on her face and stirred the food around her plate, hoping her academic peers wouldn't notice, distracted by masculine conversation and a heavy meal.

Maybe a cup of tea would sooth the rumbling in her stomach until she could make a graceful exit.

> For I can do everything through Christ, who gives me strength.
> (Philippians 4:13 NLT)

Prayer: Lord, when I feel as though I just can't make it through the next few minutes or hours, please give me the strength to hold on and accomplish all that you have called me to do.

Chapter 31

HELPFUL HINTS: MANAGING NAUSEA

1. Take the anti-nausea medication as prescribed. You may want to take the meds thirty to forty-five minutes prior to a meal. If the medicine is ineffective, notify your doctor.

2. Avoid spicy, greasy, or rich foods.

3. Keep a supply of crackers, toast, pudding, gelatin, white soda, chicken noodle soup, mashed potatoes, and other bland foods on hand.

4. Try flat warm soda if fizzy drinks cause nausea.

5. If the odors of hot foods make you nauseated, stick with cold foods.

6. Prepare in advance those foods that usually appeal to you when you experience flu-like symptoms.

7. Eat several small meals throughout the day.

8. Stay hydrated. Sip liquids: flat soda, clear juices, popsicles, broth, and tea. Try flavored gelatin.

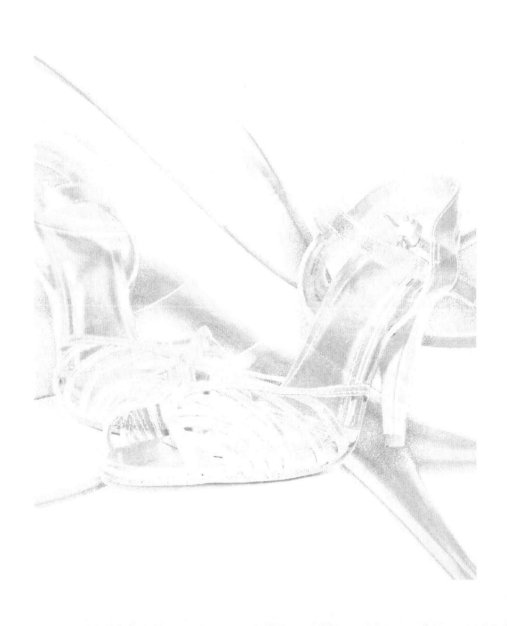

Chapter 32

Just Do It

"Tell me what I have to do," Cathie said. "I'll take care of it. Then I can get on with my life."

"You have stage one non-Hodgkin's lymphoma," the oncologist said. "Your treatment will include several months of chemotherapy followed by radiotherapy. Within two weeks of chemo, you will lose all of your hair."

Cathie drove herself nearly an hour and a half each way to receive chemotherapy every third Friday. To avoid missing work, she snagged her doctor's last appointment of the day. She planned to recover from her treatment over the weekend at home. When radiotherapy started, she requested a daily seven o'clock a.m. appointment, so she could drive straight from her treatment to work. She didn't want to be late for school.

She had completed her first round of chemotherapy when she accepted an invitation to a pool party at a friend's home. The day of the party, Cathie woke to find strands of hair strewn across her pillow. Hair littered the vanity and clung to her comb and fingertips. She grabbed the hairspray and sprayed what was left of her short crop of hair, nearly emptying the can. *Not one hair will be allowed to drop from my head today!* After a last triumphant glance in the mirror, she grabbed her purse and headed to the party.

"My mom's hair didn't fall out from chemo," Cathie's friend said. "I'll bet your hair won't fall out either."

"Bet me a new shirt?" Cathie asked. Later that month, Cathie whipped off her hat and modeled her bald head for her friend.

"I guess I owe you a new top," her friend said.

The Sunday after Cathie's second chemotherapy treatment, she developed a fever. She called in sick for work Monday morning. This was her only sick day due to cancer. She drove to the clinic to have her labs drawn and discovered her red blood cell and white blood cell counts had dropped due to the chemotherapy.

She started on a set of injections designed to increase her blood counts. One injection was prescribed daily. A nurse friend of hers volunteered to give her the injections. Every day before work, she stopped by her friend's home to receive her medication.

As the school principal, Cathie felt that wearing a wig would be more professional than the hats she wore at home to shield her boys from the reality of cancer.

During one of her chemotherapy treatments after work, Cathie's nurse said, "I like your hair."

"It's a wig," she said.

"I know," the nurse replied.

Cathie glanced around the room, noting that most of the women surrounding her still possessed their own hair. "Am I missing something here?" Cathie asked her nurse. "Is it the shampoo or the conditioner? Is there some product I should be using on my head?"

"No, Cathie. Their chemo is not as harsh as yours."

Despite her treatments, Cathie strove to make life as normal as possible for her boys. While on the way to her sons' basketball game, gusts of wind whipped the bare tree branches.

"Mom, it's really windy out," one of her sons said.

Another piped in, "We're afraid your wig is going to blow off your head!"

"Ok, guys," Cathie said. "You walk in first, and I'll walk in a little later so if my hair does blow off, you won't be embarrassed."

Cathie's hair grew back kinky and mousy gray. One day, she grabbed her wig and dashed into the salon. "I want this color," she said, tugging the one-half inch of gray hair. "To be this color." She waved the wig under her hairdresser's nose.

Her hairdresser selected a hair dye and squirted the contents of the bottle on Cathie's head, massaging the color into her gray bristles. After washing and blow-drying her hair, she swung Cathie around in the chair to face the mirror.

"Perfect!" Cathie ditched her wig.

The next day at school, a student said, "Hey, Mrs. C., why did you cut your hair so short?"

Another chimed in, "It's ok, you still look beautiful, Mrs. C."

The K-5 students had been oblivious to her medical condition. Mission accomplished.

She promised her students if they read a certain number of books by the end of the school year, she would kiss a pig.

They enthusiastically complied. Since this had been Cathie's first year as a school principal, a local newspaper featured an article touting the reading activity of her students. On the front page, they splashed a picture of Cathie sporting her wig—kissing a pig.

> And let us run with perseverance the race marked out for us. (Hebrews 12:1b NIV)

Prayer: Lord, I am running a race not of my own choosing. Please help me to persevere and finish well. Help me to just do it.

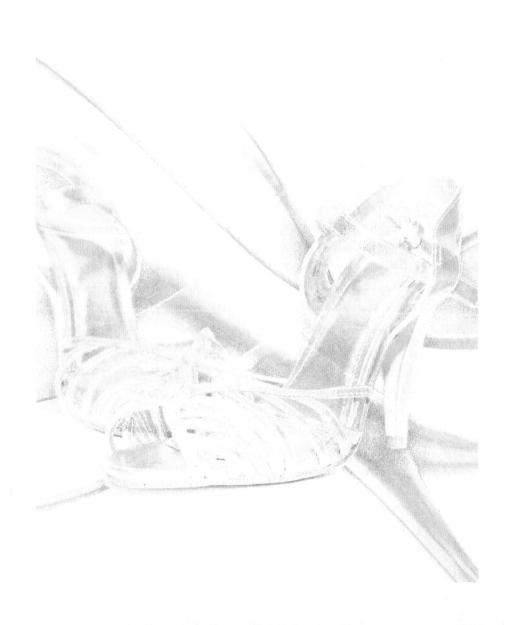

Part 3

Jill: Ovarian Cancer

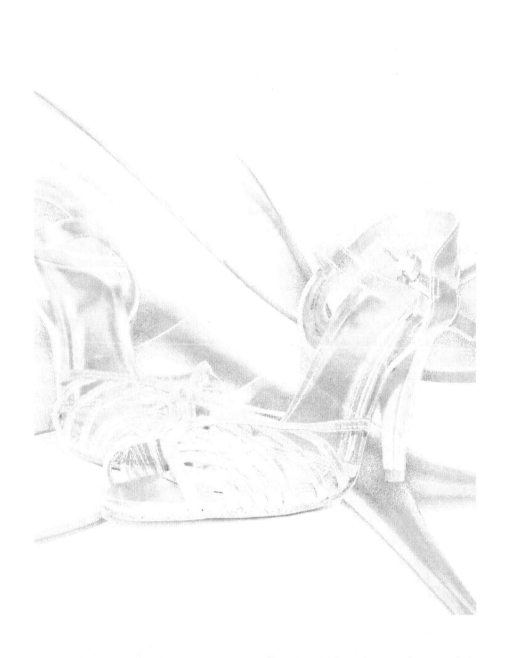

Chapter 33

SUMMER RIVALS

For Jill, summer was supposed to be crammed with swim meets—the sounds of whistles and splashes, the pungent odor of chlorine, and the invigorating challenge of rivals. A champion swimmer, she juggled two swim teams and took on a schedule that had once energized her in hopes of winning trophies and breaking records. But lately, thirteen-year-old Jill slept between practices and meets. She experienced bouts of fatigue, abdominal bloating, nausea, and vomiting. Still, she broke the all-city record in the fifty-meter backstroke.

According to her doctor, an irritable bowel caused her gastrointestinal distress, so she ignored her symptoms, as did her doctor.

After an orthodontist appointment one sultry afternoon, Jill's sister dropped her off at the food court in the mall to wait for their mom. Feeling queasy, Jill propped herself up against the door and rubbed her distended belly. She wished her mom would hurry up and get off work.

Jill spotted her mom. *Why is she looking at me like that?* Mom's wide-eyed stare hadn't gone unnoticed by Jill. Her Umbro shorts and baggy shirt couldn't hide her swollen belly, which had expanded overnight and resembled a full-term pregnancy.

Fearing hemorrhage, Mom rushed Jill to the pediatrician, then on to the hospital for an emergency ultrasound.

In the dim room, the ultrasound technician squeezed cold gel on Jill's bloated abdomen and pressed the probe across her taut skin.

Jill winced.

Partway through the exam, the tech excused herself and returned with an entourage of medical personnel. They jockeyed for position to catch a glimpse of the image appearing on the ultrasound screen.

The primary doctor diagnosed a ruptured tumor and prepared Jill and her parents for the upcoming surgery.

Jill glanced at her parents and then at her doctor. *They all seem so calm. I guess there's nothing to worry about. Everything will be all right.*

Jill had yet to grasp that a new rival had emerged—ovarian cancer.

> But I have calmed and quieted myself, I am like a weaned child with its mother; like a weaned child I am content. (Psalm 131:2 NIV)

Prayer: Thank you, Lord, for calming me when I face circumstances that I don't understand.

Chapter 34

WISPIES

Jill raked her hand through her thinning hair. Silky wisps clung to her fingers. She laughed as she thrust her arm through the open window of the moving vehicle. The rippling breeze snagged the wisps, scattering them aloft over the city like ashes from an urn. Drama in the life of a normal thirteen-year-old girl was supposed to revolve around sports, boys, fashion, and makeup. The manual of puberty neglected to include a chapter entitled "Chemotherapy-Induced Baldness."

Earlier that day, Jill arrived at the theater for a matinee showing of *Casper* with her mom and her grandparents.

Grandma's eyes widened, mesmerized by the expanse of the screen. "My, look at that!"

Mom and Jill locked glances, rolling their eyes and shaking their heads, grateful for the sparsely filled seats. Oohs and aahs gushed from her grandparents' lips as a cartoon Casper spiraled in flight through the actors' bodies of flesh

Embarrassed by her grandparents' outbursts, Jill sank her six-foot frame deeper into the plush chair, staring straight ahead at the screen. To amuse herself, she combed her fingers through her hair, allowing the feathery wisps to float onto the coke-stained floor. After the movie, Jill raced out of the theater without a backward glance at her grandparents or the pile of hair tucked under her seat. Her destination—a gummy bear parfait treat.

Even as wisps increasingly replaced her chestnut locks, Jill resisted the pressure to shave her head. The hole in the back of her baseball cap corralled the wisps, hiding the bald spot and gave her confidence. She determined that no one would see her bald head, including her family.

The one person Jill couldn't hide her baldness from was herself. The loss of her wavy tresses provoked frequent outbursts of tears. One particularly weepy day, Jill steered her IV pole down the hall of the pediatric oncology unit. Bald-headed children surrounded her, a constant reminder of her own heartbreak.

A young man spun by in a wheelchair. Only one leg protruded from beneath his hospital gown. Mom reminded Jill that her hair would grow back, but this boy's leg would not.

Mom had established a new perspective for Jill's baldness. Her hair loss and grief would be temporary.

> But I will restore you to health and heal your wounds. (Jeremiah 30:17 NLT)

Prayer: Thank you, Lord, for your promise to restore what I lost and for showing me your perspective.

Chapter 35

The Trophy

While Jill lay in the hospital hooked up to machines pumping chemotherapy into her veins, her teammates hit the water at the Phillips 66 National Swimming Championships. For Jill, all hopes of championship medals were crushed. This meet, the highlight of the year, would qualify the next US Olympic swim team for the Atlanta games.

Jill's coach had escorted his Olympic hopefuls to the championships. Anticipation of trophies and medals mounted, but his thoughts strayed back to his benched swimmer. He had an idea. He grabbed a white swim cap, embossed with the meet's logo—the American flag. Between the blast of the buzzer and the roar of the crowds, he dashed around the pool, asking the swimmers—including some of the newly qualified Olympians—to autograph the cap. Sympathetic to Jill, they gladly complied.

Due to Coach's phobia of hospitals, he stashed the swim cap until Jill returned home from her chemotherapy hospitalization. Wringing the swim cap in his hands, he rang the doorbell.

Jill cracked the door, wisps of hair peeking out from underneath her baseball cap. As he offered her the swim cap, he shuffled his feet and stammered out the tale surrounding the cap.

She clasped the outstretched cap, caressing each signature. The gleam in her eyes registered her thanks.

Jill's favorite swimmer and role model, Amy Van Dyken, had autographed the swim cap. She identified with Amy. Both girls, each six-foot tall, sported shoulder-length chestnut hair and shared a medical history of asthma. In the

Atlanta Olympics, Amy pressed on and made history as the first American female athlete to win four gold medals in a single Olympic game.

God had not forgotten a thirteen-year-old girl compelled to replace competitions with chemotherapy. Jill received the best trophy of all—the autographed stars and stripes swim cap. She hung the treasure, framed in glass, in a place of honor above all her other trophies. She never forgot her coach, who, despite his terror of hospitals, interrupted his hectic schedule to remember one of his own.

> Every good and perfect gift is from above, coming down from the Father. (James 1:17 NIV)

Prayer: Lord, I'm amazed that you know exactly what I need to cheer me up. Thank you for your delightful surprises in the midst of my suffering. Open my eyes to see the good gifts you've given me.

Chapter 36

FURRY BUDDIES

Jill stretched her long arms across the top bunk of her bed, too weak to climb the ladder. She scooped up her stuffed animals and crammed them into her athletic bag. After rearranging wisps of hair under her University of Michigan baseball cap, she lugged her bag to the car. Another round of chemotherapy at Children's Hospital.

Hugging her bear to her chest, Jill buried her face in his plush fur. MAC Bear, a gift from the Madison Aquatics Club came complete with a miniature club T-shirt and swim goggles. He reminded her of their love and support as well as her life before cancer. He never left her side. By day, he provided constant companionship while she sprawled on the couch, eyes glued to the O.J. Simpson trial and the reruns of *Quantum Leap*. By night, MAC Bear lay curled in her arms.

Smiley face balloons, color drawings, toys, and stuffed animals personalized the children's hospital rooms. Jill hung the smaller stuffed animals on her IV pole that secured her chemotherapy pump. Her collection included Polar Bear, Jeff the black bear, and Orangutan, who doubled as a wrist support for her IV hand after surgery.

Satisfied, she stepped back and admired her handiwork. One, two, three … she counted her hanging critters. Oh, no! Thirteen! Thirteen—an unlucky number. Thirteen—her age when diagnosed with cancer. Jill scoured through her bag and bedding for another furry friend.

A knock at the door interrupted her panicked search. The Child Life coordinator stepped in. Sympathetic to Jill's unlucky thirteen, she scavenged for another stuffed animal. Success! She presented Jill with Pink Piggy.

Grinning her thanks, Jill added Pink Piggy to her IV pole menagerie. Fourteen. Even MAC bear appeared relieved, resting against her pillow.

And my God shall supply all your need according to His riches in glory by Christ Jesus. (Philippians 4:19 NKJV)

Prayer: Lord, some may consider my requests silly, but you never take lightly that which you know is important to me. Thank you for answering my seemingly insignificant prayers in tangible ways.

Chapter 37

A Child's Eye View

Jill lay in her hospital bed snuggling MAC Bear as chemotherapy dripped into her veins, Mom stationed by her side. Startled by a knock at the door, Jill opened her eyes to see a long, black robe swishing over shiny black shoes. Her gaze followed the robe up the towering figure and rested on the starched white collar that brushed his wrinkled throat.

After his initial greeting, the chaplain moved toward Jill and said with a solemn voice, "Let's pray."

Jill's eyes widened in horror as the black-clad pastor drew near. Ministers in black meant last rites and funerals. *No one told me I'm going to die! Is my funeral next? It's just a tumor!* White knuckled, Jill clasped her mom's arm. She looked at Mom pleadingly.

Mom pulled away from her daughter's grip and escorted the minister to the door. She suggested he not return.

Jill trembled as she clutched MAC Bear to her chest. Tears trickled down her pale cheeks.

Mom slid onto the bed, laying her hand on her daughter's quivering shoulder and reassured her that she was not going to die. In a few months, she would be back in school and competing in swim meets.

Jill wiped her eyes. Mom wouldn't lie.

On another day, Jill's gynecologic oncologist planned a consultation during evening rounds with her and her family. The visit coincided with dinnertime. Since the smell of hospital food gagged her, the Child Life coordinator had supplied meal tickets for the cafeteria. With frequent glances at the clock, Jill and Mom waited. *How much longer?* The cafeteria would soon close, and Jill would get crabby if she ate late.

By the time her physician arrived two hours later, Jill's crankiness had escalated.

She ripped into the doctor, accusing him of being rude and inconsiderate. After all, common courtesy required a phone call if one expected to be late. Moreover, the cafeteria had closed. She'd missed dinner.

After this, the doctor shifted Jill to the front of his rounds. He was never late again. Her mom later told her she had silently cheered for her.

Ovarian cancer thrust Jill into the world of adult oncology. The hospital boasted a kid-friendly environment, but once in a while, the multiple team members forgot that this six-foot teenager was still a child. They missed the view from a child's eyes.

> And whoever welcomes one such child in my name welcomes me.
> (Matthew 18:5 NIV)

Prayer: Lord, sometimes the people who should understand the most seem blind to my troubles. Thank you, Lord, that you understand me.

Chapter 38

Kid-Friendly

Jill clutched MAC Bear as she walked down the corridors of Children's Hospital, dodging Red Flyer wagons and wheelchairs. Murals of carefree kids lined the walls, beckoning a path to the oncology wing. Anchored by stuffed animals, smiley face balloons swayed as they peered through open doorways. A schoolroom, playroom, and even a teen room stocked with video games lined an adjacent hallway. In this kid-friendly zone, freezers crammed with popsicles and ice cream were quickly depleted, sticky fingerprints left all around the room.

One evening, Jill had reserved the TV lounge for a movie night. Her anticipation mounted as the beverages chilled. The smell of buttery popcorn permeated the room, luring her friends. With her baseball cap pulled over her eyes, she sauntered down the hall. Stuffed animals swung from her IV pole while chemotherapy pumped into her veins.

Rowdy teenagers crowded around the TV/VCR donated by former supermodel, Cindy Crawford. They popped in *Cool Runnings*, a comedy loosely based on the four-man Jamaican bobsled team that competed in the 1988 Calgary Olympics. Unfamiliar with snow, these sprinters navigated the precarious course on a borrowed bobsled, finishing last. The kids' laughter echoed down the antiseptic corridors as the team's misadventures provided a welcome distraction from the reality of cancer.

Jill's surgeon never forgot that Jill was still a child. For Halloween, she outfitted her with a set of surgical scrubs, complete with a surgical cap to cover her bald head. The doctor included her in the consultations with her parents, acknowledging her questions and comments. When her lower lip quivered and her eyes teared due to impending procedures, her surgeon suggested alternative, less invasive tests, relieving Jill's anxiety.

Everything is about the child in the kid-friendly zone.

> Then he took the children in his arms and placed his hands on their heads and blessed them. (Mark 10:16 NLT)

Prayer: Thank you, Lord, for the safe places you provide for me, so I won't be so afraid when I am sick.

Chapter 39

BACK ON TRACK

Jill completed her chemotherapy and was ready to return to the classroom. Since wearing hats in class violated school rules, Jill received special permission to wear baseball caps until her hair grew back.

During student council registration, she donned her Umbro shorts, a baggy shirt, and her favorite University of Michigan baseball cap. A fellow student mistook her for a boy, with her lanky six-foot frame and cap. She crossed her arms and glared at him, tears pooling in her eyes.

One month after chemotherapy ended, Jill resumed swimming. She looked forward to her familiar practice schedule. The pungent odor of chlorine and gym shoes permeated the locker room. Self-conscious of her baldness, she waited for all of the other swimmers to enter the pool. She peeked around the corner. With one sweep of her hand, she knocked off her baseball hat and slid her swim cap over her bald head then joined her teammates. No one would see her bald.

In time, crocuses and tulips replaced the snow, signaling not only the arrival of spring but track and field season also. Swimming had strengthened Jill's shoulder muscles for the discus throw. During practice, one of the boys snuck up behind her and whipped off her cap as she pivoted and hurled the discus. With her free hand, she reached for her hat.

Too late. Mortified, tears stung her eyes as she shielded her bald head with her long arms. The remorseful prankster thrust the cap into her hand and mumbled an apology as he backed away.

Since the loss of her hair, Jill had avoided mirrors. But the anticipation of new hair growth drew her back to the mirror like a magnet. Her hope for blonde hair was stamped "Denied" when dark Brillo Pad stubble sprouted between the wisps. No matter. Soon, short waves replaced the bristles, and Jill triumphantly clipped off her wispies.

Now her life had returned to normal. She was back on track.

> Though I walk in the midst of trouble, you preserve my life.
> (Psalm 138:7 NIV)

Prayer: Lord, this has been such a difficult season for me, grieving the loss of my hair, my self-image, and my familiar routine. Thank you for your faithfulness, for restoring my life, and for guiding me through this time.

Part 4

Joanne: Breast Cancer

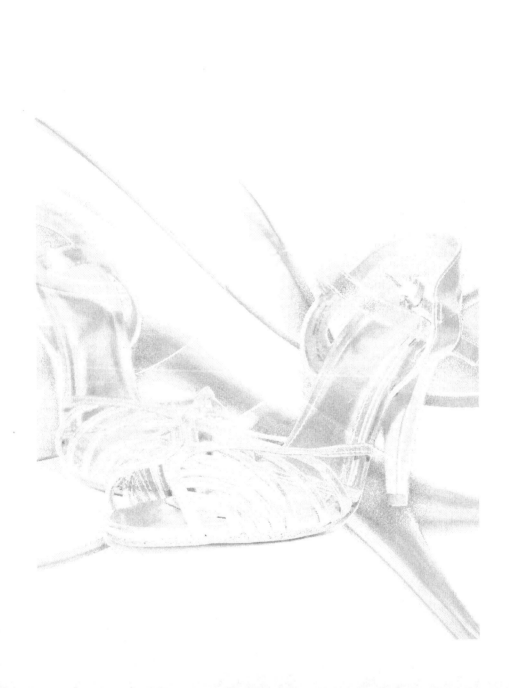

Chapter 40

NOT AGAIN!

"This just isn't fair after all we've been through," Joanne cried as she flung herself into her husband's arms.

Almost a year had passed since their thirteen-year-old daughter, Jill, had undergone surgery and chemotherapy for ovarian cancer.

That afternoon, a phone call had interrupted her workday with the results of her breast biopsy. Stunned, Joanne walked into the break room and calmly announced to her friend, "I have breast cancer."

Several weeks earlier, while performing a self-breast exam, Joanne had discovered a lump. The physician's assistant didn't believe the cyst was malignant, but Joanne insisted on a biopsy. During the procedure, a sinking feeling gripped her as she glanced at the doctor's face, partially hidden by his surgical mask.

His brow furrowed in an unspoken message—cancer. The doctor reassured her the mass was small and treatable, but she needed a lymph node biopsy.

After composing herself, she punched in the numbers for the dreaded phone call. "Mom, I have breast cancer."

A piercing wail resounded from the other end of the line.

Joanne rushed to reassure her. "Mom, I've dealt with cancer for a year now with Jill, and I refuse to allow it to consume our lives any longer."

Memories of Jill's hospitalizations and chemotherapy flooded Joanne's mind: weakness, nausea, and hair loss, as well as her own fear and exhaustion. Juggling two careers and two daughters had drained their parental strength.

Her husband had worked afternoons, caring for Jill in the morning. Joanne spent mornings in the office, then drove straight to the hospital to be by her daughter's side until nightfall. Under a veil of darkness, Joanne would drive home, her vision clouded by tears.

They refused to neglect their older daughter or miss her swim meets. Joanne cheered her on during the home meets while her husband traveled to the out-of-town meets. Cancer had devastated and disrupted their lives once, and Joanne resolved that cancer would not have that power again.

> Into your hands I commit my spirit; deliver me, Lord, my faithful God. (Psalm 31:5 NIV)

Prayer: Lord, I thank you that cancer does not rule my life. I put my life in your hands.

Chapter 41

DOES ANYONE HEAR ME?

After her lumpectomy for breast cancer, Joanne vomited repeatedly, sick from anesthesia. She was unable to even keep water down. Her surgeon suggested she remain in the hospital overnight. Exhausted from retching and numerous treks to the bathroom, Joanne gratefully accepted. She glanced at her reflection in the mirror. Green-tinged skin encircled her sunken eyes. Thankfully, her girls had competed in swim meets this evening. She didn't want them to see her so ill.

"Time to go home!" the nurse's voice boomed out as she rolled a wheelchair into the room.

Joanne mumbled from the bowels of the bathroom between dry heaves, "I don't think I can make the drive home without throwing up." *Didn't the doctor say I could stay?*

"You'll be fine." the nurse replied. "I'll give you a bag." She stripped the bed with such force, she nearly ripped the sheets.

She plopped Joanne into a wheelchair and shoved a barf bag into her hand. As if on cue, Joanne threw up. In her weakened state, she hoped her husband would stand up for her and reiterate their conversation with the doctor.

Instead, he awkwardly stood by, bamboozled by anything medical. Oblivious to her distress, he grabbed the wheelchair bearing his wife slumped over her paper bag. Per the nurse's orders, he wheeled her out of the hospital.

The next morning, the surgeon called their home. Concerned, he asked why they'd left the hospital when he'd written orders for her to stay overnight. Joanne fumed as she related the previous day's events, unsure of who she was most angry with—the nurse or her husband. Yes, she assured the doctor, she was all right. That morning she was able to keep down a little dry toast and tea.

Later in the day, she received an apologetic phone call from the nursing supervisor. *That nurse deserves whatever trouble she got herself into.*

Still traumatized, Joanne was determined that no future grandchild would carry the name of that nurse.

> The LORD himself goes before you and will be with you; he will
> never leave you nor forsake you. (Deuteronomy 31:8 NIV)

Prayer: Father, sometimes I feel so alone with no one to fight for me. Thank you, Lord, that even when others haven't stood up for me or helped me, you never leave me alone or desert me.

Chapter 42

DREAMS COME TRUE

After looking over Joanne's biopsy results, the doctor discussed her radiotherapy treatment for breast cancer.

"I have to host a spaghetti dinner for the whole swim team," Joanne said. "I won't allow these treatments to interfere with the dinner or with my daughters' major swim meets."

Taken aback, the doctor agreed to schedule the treatments on her terms.

Joanne refused to allow her girls to be traumatized again by cancer. Maintaining a positive attitude, she said to her daughters, "I just need to go through a few weeks of radiation therapy, and then I'll be fine."

To dispel their fears, Joanne invited her daughters to accompany her to a five-minute radiotherapy treatment. Her treatment was quick and pain-free. Joanne was relieved when her girls relaxed and slipped back into their normal behavior patterns.

After five weeks of radiotherapy, Joanne received her last treatment two days before Christmas—her best Christmas present ever. Enough of doctors and clinics. Despite the "what ifs" toying with her mind, she had no time to feel sorry for herself. She would set sail on a new course. Family vacations, graduation parties, and the joys of life unfurled before her.

As the years passed, Joanne clapped and cheered while her girls marched with honors to "Pomp and Circumstance." Joy burst forth from her heart when her daughters, arrayed in beaded satin, glided down the aisle on their father's tuxedoed arm.

On Jill's wedding day, Joanne's misty eyes lingered on her daughter as she twirled around the dance floor in the arms of her groom. "There was a time I never thought I would see this day," she whispered.

Hope deferred makes the heart sick, but a dream fulfilled is a tree of life. (Proverbs 13:12 NLT)

Prayer: Lord, I've been through some really hard days I didn't think I'd survive. Thank you for pulling me through and enabling me to live to see the fulfillment of not only my hopes and dreams but also those of my children.

Chapter 43

CONFIDENCE CRUSHED

Joanne approached her mammogram with an unusual air of confidence. Normally, her worry meter would've matched the heat of that July Monday.

"You've gone fifteen years with no recurrence," her oncologist had said during Joanne's appointment the previous summer. "I'm going to release you from my care. Call me if you have any further problems."

With her mammogram behind her, Joanne drove ninety miles the next day to be with her dad. Grief over the loss of his wife fourteen months earlier hindered him from handling his financial affairs. Every Tuesday, father and daughter hit the casino, followed by lunch, the grocery store then back to the house so Joanne could pay his bills.

Amid the ching-ching of the slot machines, Joanne's phone chimed. Immediately, she recognized the clinic's number. Pressing the phone to her ear, she scurried out of the casino, straining to catch the clinician's words. The din of boisterous conversations and blaring music followed her, spilled into the lobby, and drowned out the voice on the other end of the line. She headed outside, shielding her eyes from the sunlight.

"We need to repeat your mammogram and perform an ultrasound," the radiologist said. "We think the breast cancer has returned."

The doctor's report punched her in the gut. After she regained her composure, she wandered back into the casino to find her dad. *I can't tell my dad anything until I know for sure.*

Joanne never felt the lump. The doctor even said the growth didn't feel like cancer, but they would do a biopsy and send the tissue to pathology. Once she consulted with surgery and oncology, they formulated a plan—a lumpectomy with a lymph node biopsy.

Once the biopsy results arrived, the oncologist laid out her course of treatment. "You'll have a total of eight rounds of chemotherapy, one month off and then six and a half weeks of radiation. We'll place a port beneath the skin in your chest to infuse the chemotherapy, since the drugs will be too harsh for your peripheral veins." The doctor continued, attempting to reassure her, "Even though the cancer is aggressive, it tends to respond well to chemotherapy."

Joanne and her husband took a drive with her dad after she completed all of her appointments. "Dad, the cancer is back," she said and laid out her course of treatment.

"This hasn't been a very good year for us," he said.

Joanne agreed. She had determined the treatment would deliver the promised results. Next year would be better.

> For you have been my hope, Sovereign LORD, my confidence since my youth. (Psalm 71:5 NIV)

Prayer: Lord, thank you that I can place my confidence in you and in your unfailing love, even when my life seems to be unraveling around me.

Chapter 44

RESEARCH, RESEARCH, RESEARCH

Cancer had spun her life out of control once again, but Joanne knew, armed with information, she could cope and maintain some semblance of order. She surfed the internet for the most up-to-date breast cancer treatments and symptom management. The information spawned lists of questions, which she addressed with her oncologist.

She found neuropathies to be one of the most disturbing side effects. She knew women who suffered with debilitating numbness of the hands and feet, persisting long after chemotherapy. Breast cancer blogs posted tips and preventative antidotes. Joanne printed out the information and handed the papers to her doctor, who was willing to try these alternative remedies.

One treatment involved wrapping cooling mats around the hands and feet during chemotherapy. The therapy was based on the premise that the cold would constrict the blood vessels and prevent the chemotherapy from affecting the extremities. Since Joanne couldn't find cooling mats, she brought dishpans to her treatments and filled them with ice water. Every twenty minutes during her four-hour chemotherapy treatment, she submerged her hands and feet in the ice water for ten to fifteen minutes. The technique worked until after the fourth treatment.

Five days later, her feet felt numb.

Her fingers didn't escape the attack of neuropathy either. The effects lasted several days after each treatment. Not only did fatigue make doing laundry difficult, but the increased sensitivity in her fingertips made the task downright painful. When she unscrewed the cap of the laundry detergent bottle, pain shot through her fingertips as if someone grabbed her fingernails and ripped them off.

The pain in Joanne's fingertips resolved after chemotherapy, but the numbness in her heels and in the balls of her feet persisted. While descending the stairs, she continued to grab hold of the rail. Her heel tended to catch on the edge of the stair since she couldn't feel her foot landing on the step. She found comfort in knowing she'd tried her best to minimize the neuropathy.

> So I turned my mind to understand, to investigate and to search out wisdom. (Ecclesiastes 7:25 NIV)

Prayer: Lord, I have so much information available at my fingertips today. Please give me wisdom as I search for instruction and guide me to those things that would be helpful.

Chapter 45

SAFEGUARDS

Joanne carefully pored over the chemotherapy information and instruction pamphlets given to her in the oncology clinic. Some of the material proved to be unsettling.

She discovered the chemotherapy drugs could be secreted in her body fluids for about forty-eight hours after each treatment. Joanne would need to safeguard her family.

She religiously wiped the toilet seat and flushed the toilet twice after each use as instructed and carefully washed her hands with soap and water, using only paper towels to dry. After eating, she thoroughly washed her own dishes and flatware, even before placing them in the dishwasher.

Managing her environment was the easy part. But how would she explain to her grandchild that she couldn't sit on grandma's lap? The doctor said the chemotherapy would probably be out of her system toward the end of each treatment, so contact should be safe. *Should* … But Joanne's research indicated that her chemotherapy drugs could remain in her system for up to a month. She wouldn't take any chances.

One month after her first chemotherapy treatment, Joanne's youngest daughter presented her with a grandson. Excited, Joanne visited them in the hospital and posed for his newborn pictures, but her husband held this bundle of joy. She refrained from stroking his downy hair and playing with his tiny fingers and toes. As much as she would've loved to hold her new grandson, the risk wasn't worth exposing the baby to any residual chemotherapy.

One month after her last chemotherapy treatment, Grandma Joanne proudly cuddled her new grandson. At four and one-half months old, he was worth the wait. She'd done her best to keep her family safe.

You, LORD, will keep the needy safe and will protect us. (Psalm 12:7 NIV)

Prayer: Lord, I've done all I know to do to protect my loved ones, but ultimately, I rely on you to protect us and keep us safe.

Chapter 46

Mirror, Mirror on the Wall

Joanne stockpiled scarves and wigs when she learned that chemotherapy threatened to strip away her hair. Accompanied by a friend, she arrived at her appointment to select her first wig. The stylist chose an ash-colored hairpiece and held it up to Joanne.

"No," Joanne said. This was no match for her brunette coloring.

"How about chin length?" the stylist said.

"No, that was the style I wore when I was thirty," Joanne replied. She finally settled on a wig that matched her current cut and color.

When her hair started to fall out, she asked her beautician to shave her head. She had faithfully practiced the art of scarf tying in preparation for this day, so she grabbed her wig and scarves and headed out to her appointment.

"Should I shave your hair down to a half-inch?" Joanne's hairdresser asked. This was the first time she'd shaved the head of a woman undergoing chemotherapy.

"One quarter-inch," Joanne said. Her beautician gripped the razor, tears pooling in her eyes as she tentatively grazed Joanne's scalp.

I don't want to see her cry. Joanne surveyed her shorn head in the mirror. She reached for her scarf and wrapped the fabric around her head just as she'd practiced.

When she went shopping for a second wig, she took the same friend who'd helped her the first time. Once in the shop, Joanne slipped off her wig.

Her friend drew back, wide eyed. "Oh!" Quickly, she diverted attention from her initial shock of viewing Joanne's bald head. "Do you mind if I rub your scalp?"

Joanne consented, receiving a scalp massage while she selected another wig.

Joanne could look at herself bald, but she couldn't handle her baldness being seen by another person. She waited a month before she unveiled her bald head in front of her husband. After her shower, she wrapped her head in a towel just like she did when she still had hair. A sleep cap covered her baldness at night since her head easily chilled. Sometimes, she sported a cap with bangs mimicking some semblance of normalcy. She carefully covered her head when around her grandchildren. *Would they be afraid of losing their hair from taking their medication?*

Joanne stared at her reflection in the mirror. Dark shadows circled her eyes, framed by a sallow complexion. "You really do look terrible, don't you?" she said. Then she laughed. No matter how bad she felt, she showered, applied her make-up and penciled in her eyebrows. Tying a fashionable scarf around her head, she completed her morning routine. If she looked good, then maybe she would feel better.

> You are altogether beautiful, my darling; there is no flaw in you.
> (Song of Songs 4:7 NIV)

Prayer: Lord, sometimes when I see my reflection in the mirror, I have a hard time overlooking the flaws. Thank you that no matter how I view myself, you still see me as beautiful.

Chapter 47

GAME DAY

Game day. Just enough time for Joanne and her husband to grab a bite to eat before the Big Ten football game. They slipped on their red team sweatshirts and headed out to the restaurant. On the way, pain squeezed Joanne's sternum, snatching her breath. She clutched her chest, but the vice-like grip held secure. Her jaw ached. *Am I having a heart attack?*

She dug around in her purse until she latched on to her cell phone. Between puffed breaths, she called the oncologist.

"I think your chest pain is probably bone pain, a side effect of your chemotherapy," the doctor said. "But I want you to go to the emergency room and have them check you over."

In the emergency room, the nurses inserted the oxygen prongs into Joanne's nose, stuck the cardiac patches on her chest, and hooked her up to the monitor. The technician rolled in the ECG machine while the nurse drew blood samples from her chemotherapy port.

The medical staff fired off questions in rapid succession.

"No, I've never had this pain before," Joanne answered. "No, I'm not nauseated, dizzy, or short of breath. No, I don't have any history of heart disease."

Once the staff completed the initial tests and medicated her for pain, the emergency room hustle and bustle shifted to the adjacent cubicles. Relegated to waiting mode, Joanne and her husband cheered their favorite team to victory via the television screen. With Joanne propped up on an emergency room cart and her husband perched on a straight-back chair, they occupied the most expensive game seats in the house. Hour by hour the clock ticked, the long-awaited supper kicked to the wayside.

The doctor discharged her after eight hours of emergency room hospitality and game-side seating. Despite the scare, Joanne had not suffered a heart attack. The doctors concluded that the ache in her sternum was due to chemotherapy. They assured her she had done the right thing coming into the emergency room to have the chest pain evaluated.

Even though the doctor told her that her joints might ache, no one had prepared Joanne for stabbing chest pain that mimicked a heart attack. The bone pain resolved after she completed her chemotherapy treatments.

> My health may fail, and my spirit may grow weak, but God remains the strength of my heart; he is mine forever. (Psalm 73:26 NLT)

Prayer: Lord, sometimes the side effects of chemotherapy scare me. Thank you for providing the help I so desperately need.

Chapter 48

INFLAMED

Breakfast—the morning challenge. What was she going to eat? Joanne opened the cabinet and scanned the cereal line-up. Corn flakes. Granola. Their sharp, irregular-shaped pieces tore at the sores lining the inside of her mouth and throat. Even buttered toast cut like ground glass. So once again, she vacillated between grits and oatmeal, cooled in a sea of milk.

Thirty minutes before her soft, bland meal, she swished the magic mouthwash around in her mouth before swallowing. Magic because the liquid included an oral anesthetic. No morning coffee. Hot liquids and acidic food burned her sensitive palate as if she had gargled with boiling water. She dipped her finger into her tea. Lukewarm, the perfect temperature.

Joanne slid her tongue over the roof of her mouth. Peeling skin like sunburn caught the tip of her tongue. She tried to examine the sores in the mirror, but since opening her mouth hurt, she couldn't visualize any of the ulcerations. Toward the end of her chemotherapy cycle, she experienced several days of improvement in the severity of the mouth sores. But her next treatment once again kick-started the tormenting sting.

Spicy food fired up the heat and pain in her mouth. No snacking on chips and salsa. Boxes of cherry-flavored popsicles lined Joanne's freezer. Their cold nectar soothed her raw mouth and throat.

On a good day, Joanne's husband took her out to their favorite fast-food restaurant. Usually health-conscious, Joanne shuddered at the thought of eating French fries, but during her chemotherapy treatments, they actually tasted normal, a rarity those days. She waited for her hamburger and fries to cool and then ripped them into tiny pieces before eating. A treat of frozen custard soothed the throat irritation stirred up by her meal.

About four weeks after the chemotherapy ended, the mouth sores disappeared. Joanne was relieved. Fruit, soups, and smoothies spun with Greek yogurt no longer comprised the bulk of her nutrition.

> Open your mouth wide, and I will fill it with good things. (Psalm 81:10 NLT)

Prayer: Thank you, Lord, that the mouth sores are temporary, and that you provide food I can eat and medicine to help me cope with the pain.

Chapter 49

HELPFUL HINTS: MANAGING MOUTH SORES

1. Use a soft-bristled toothbrush, using toothpaste for sensitive teeth. Gently floss daily. If you have open sores in your mouth, a toothbrush may be too painful. Instead, try some mouth swabs dipped in water. Avoid lemon glycerin swabs, since they can be drying. Contact your doctor if you have open mouth sores or pain.

2. Avoid commercial mouthwashes since they are alcohol-based and may dry or irritate your mouth. Try a mouthwash of salt water (1 teaspoon of salt in 1 cup of warm water).

3. Eat foods cold or at room temperature. Avoid hot or warm foods.

4. Avoid acidic foods such as citrus and tomatoes.

5. Avoid salty or spicy foods.

6. Avoid scratchy foods such as popcorn, raw vegetables, nuts, and toast. Even the seeds in berries can cause irritation for some people.

7. Eat soft foods like ice cream, applesauce, mashed potatoes, oatmeal, yogurt, pudding, cottage cheese, scrambled eggs, and pureed meats and vegetables.

8. Keep your mouth moist. Sip liquids every few minutes with a straw if possible.

9. Suck on ice chips, or popsicles, and hard candy if tolerated.

10. Use a blender to make nutritious smoothies or milkshakes.

11. Ask your provider about moisturizers for your mouth and medications to relieve pain, such as a magic mouthwash mixture.

Chapter 50

PLUGGED

Tears streamed down Joanne's cheeks as she massaged her thighs. The throbbing bone pain surpassed any ache inflicted by the worst flu.

Pain pummeled her bones and hip joints for several days after chemotherapy. She gulped the anti-inflammatory pills and the prescribed narcotics in hopes of relief. But the narcotics possessed their own counterattack—constipation.

Pain gripped Joanne's bloated abdomen, a stomachache like no other. *I've hardly eaten anything. I feel like my bowel is going to rupture.* Joanne buckled as she wrapped her arms around her belly, attempting to smother the persistent cramping. Chemotherapy had paralyzed her bowel, strangling any movement. Joanne had never had constipation issues, and once again, no one had prepared her for this side effect of chemotherapy. Her medication regimen added a plethora of stool softeners, laxatives, and probiotics.

As if the abdominal pain wasn't bad enough, the constipation gave birth to hemorrhoids. Cream, wipes, and warm baths soothed the stinging and burning.

Through trial and error, Joanne managed the joint pain, constipation, and hemorrhoids. Thankfully her bowel never ruptured.

Despite exercise and a healthy diet, constipation remained an issue even after chemotherapy.

> But as for me, I am poor and needy; please hurry to my aid, O God. You are my helper and my savior; O Lord, do not delay. (Psalm 70:5 NLT)

Prayer: Thank you, Lord, for providing medications and treatments to help me with the various pains and discomforts caused by chemotherapy.

Chapter 51

HELPFUL HINTS: MANAGING CONSTIPATION

1. Contact your doctor for recommended laxatives if you are constipated.

2. Consult your doctor first in regard to the following suggestions:

   a. Try to eat foods high in fiber such as vegetables, grains, nuts, popcorn, and fruit, including prunes and apples.

   b. Drink two to three liters of water or juice per day. Warm or hot liquids like coffee or tea may help.

   c. Exercise twenty to thirty minutes per day. Many find walking helpful.

3. Call your doctor if you have abdominal pain, blood in your stool, nausea, vomiting, are unable to pass gas, have no bowel movement for three days, or any other change in bowel pattern.

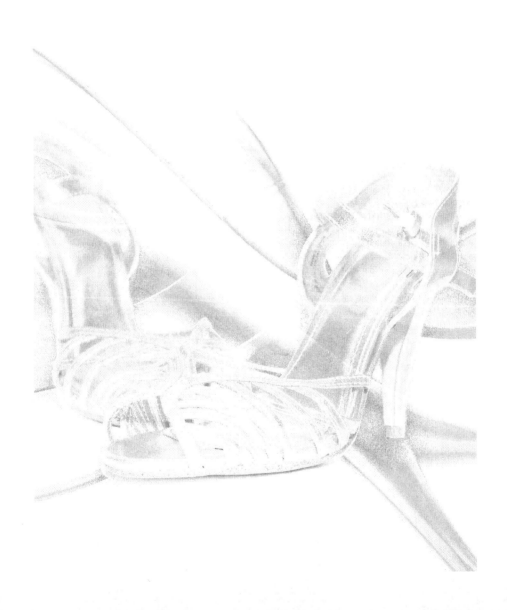

Chapter 52

A REALITY CHECK

Joanne looked forward to her vacation, even though she wasn't traveling to her usual exotic places like the Amazon or Thailand. Her doctor confined her to the mainland during her one-month hiatus between chemotherapy and radiation. Vacation destination? Florida. Joanne loved to snorkel, but she resigned herself to the fact that she would have to decline underwater exploration. Even though her mouth sores were healing, she found it difficult to hold the snorkel tube in her mouth.

When the plane landed, she grabbed her suitcase and descended the narrow stairs well ahead of her husband. Warm air fueled by the dazzling sun blasted her pale face. She strode across the tarmac, stepped through the airport door, and climbed the steps to the boarding gate.

Partway up, Joanne had to stop. She clung to the rail for support—weak and breathless.

The stewardess stationed at the boarding gate descended the narrow stairs, bumping against the oncoming passengers. "Are you all right?"

She nodded.

"Here, let me help you." She grasped Joanne's suitcase and hauled the bag the rest of the way up the steps.

Joanne pulled herself up the remaining stairs, plopped down in a seat and waited for her husband, grateful for the help. *What was I thinking? I could never have gone snorkeling.* She lamented the reality check.

She didn't realize how easily she fatigued. She thought she was past the days when she needed to sit down in the middle of the grocery aisle, space her limited activities, or forego driving.

Even though she was unable to engage in snorkeling or other activities she loved, the trip proved to be a nice break away from life on chemotherapy.

For ten days, sun, sand, and sea breezes replaced the winter chill, howling winds, and snow.

Back home, Joanne geared herself for the next phase of her treatment—radiotherapy.

> But you, LORD, do not be far from me. You are my strength; come quickly to help me. (Psalm 22:19 NIV)

Prayer: Thank you, Lord, for sending me help when my strength is small.

Chapter 53

LIVESTRONG

Joanne recalled the activities she enjoyed before chemotherapy: biking, walking, and water aerobics. Over the course of her treatment, her stamina declined. She lost confidence in her physical abilities.

After chemotherapy, she booked a trip to Italy and Greece. The extensive walking and numerous flights of stairs would challenge her endurance. She needed to jumpstart her recovery, and this trip represented the proverbial dangled carrot.

A friend of hers told her about the Livestrong program at the YMCA. Two months after completing radiotherapy, Joanne enrolled. The first meeting opened with icebreakers and allowed each member to share a little about themselves and their cancer journey. She enjoyed the small group interaction that included several other breast cancer survivors.

During those twelve weeks, personal trainers would formulate an individualized program for each of the cancer survivors to transition them from chemotherapy to normalcy.

Muscle strength, flexibility, endurance, and a healthy lifestyle comprised the goals of the Livestrong program. Personal trainers performed initial evaluations to determine baseline fitness levels and appropriate settings for the weight machines. Joanne had never exercised with machines, so the class gave her confidence to use them even while staying in hotels. The program also included a cardiovascular component. For her interval training, Joanne chose the treadmill.

The trainers encouraged their students to attend other classes offered at the YMCA. Joanne joined a silver sneakers class designed for senior citizens. Evenly spaced chairs stretched across the gym. Dumbbells, a ball, and a resistance band were stationed at each seat. To her dismay, the seniors out-performed Joanne's valiant attempts to keep up with the steps and weights.

She jumped and kicked to the high-energy music during the water-in-motion class. Spinning not only challenged her aerobically, but the hard seat poked like a burr in her backside. Even Zumba gold, tailored for seniors, had a place in the class line-up, complete with Latin music and jangling coin skirts.

The twelve-week program concluded with a lively game of wallyball—volleyball with a beach ball. A potluck not only celebrated their successes, but also marked a milestone in their quest toward a healthy lifestyle. Before departing, they shared recipes, emails, and hugs.

Livestrong propelled her toward her goal. With ease, she walked the cobblestone streets and climbed numerous flights of stairs while touring the ancient cities of Italy and Greece.

Today, Joanne still frequents the gym, continuing her program of interval and weight training as well as occasional games of pickleball. She is living strong.

He gives strength to the weary and increases the power of the weak. (Isaiah 40:29 NIV)

Prayer: Lord, I felt so discouraged by my physical weakness that prevents me from participating in the activities I love. Thank you for providing a way to restore my stamina and strength.

Part 5

Sue: Non-Hodgkin's Lymphoma

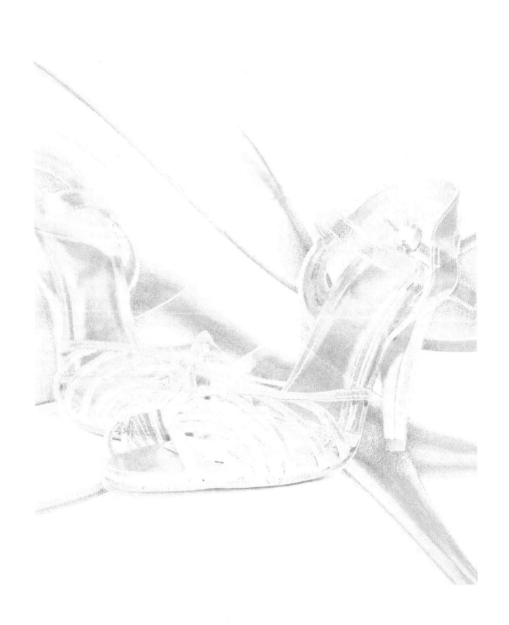

Chapter 54

CANCER? (MY ONLY VICE IS COOKIES!)

Sue grabbed the lotion, squirted a blob on her hand, and rubbed the right side of her neck. Her fingers grazed a grape-sized lump that now competed with the lump forming in her throat. *Lymphoma.* After all these years, she knew the risks. The drug she received for rheumatoid arthritis suppressed the immune system and increased her chances for developing lymphoma.

Armed with her self-diagnosis, Sue phoned her rheumatologist. Upon examination, he concluded that the swollen lymph node was just an infection. But after ten days of antibiotics, the nodule remained unchanged. With her mind still honed in on lymphoma, Sue insisted on a biopsy.

She waited all week for the surgeon to phone with the biopsy results. On Friday, she packed her girls and five of their friends for a weekend at a Country Thunder music festival. Blue skies reigned over the concert that weekend, but for Sue, dark clouds rolled in. Between performances, she phoned the surgeon's office. As far as she was concerned, he only needed to confirm her diagnosis.

"The doctor's not in," the nurse said. "He left for the weekend."

"Can you just tell me my biopsy results?" she asked.

"No, you'll have to wait until Monday when the doctor returns."

Monday morning, Sue gazed between the clock and the phone as she waited for the office to open. But the doctor refused to divulge the biopsy results until her appointment the following day. She fumed the rest of the day.

On Tuesday morning, the doctor strode into the exam room and greeted her, "How are you?"

Crossing her arms, she replied, "Well, why don't you tell me?"

"You're fine," he said.

She breathed a sigh of relief.

He continued, "You have two types of non-Hodgkin's lymphoma, one slower growing and the other more aggressive."

A scream lodged in her throat. *I am not fine!* Her subsequent CT scan revealed positive lymph nodes in her neck, groin, and ribs—non-Hodgkin's lymphoma stage III.

The doctor maintained a positive attitude as he discussed chemotherapy. Sue neglected to ask about her prognosis. To ask acknowledged the reality of cancer. *How can I have cancer? I don't smoke. I don't drink. And the only bad thing I do is eat cookies!*

> He causes his sun to rise on the evil and the good and sends rain
> on the righteous and the unrighteous. (Matthew 5:45 NIV)

Prayer: Lord, I don't understand why I have to suffer sickness when I've tried to live a good life. Please heal me and strengthen me in this season.

Chapter 55

But I Don't Have Cancer!

Ridiculous! How can I have cancer? Sue remembered how her mother-in-law had suffered from non-Hodgkin's lymphoma. Despite a remission, she died several years later from lung cancer. Was she going to have to go through all of that? She worried about her husband. As an only child, he'd been overwhelmed by his mother's deteriorating condition. Now the same disease assaulted his wife. *I'm not putting him through that again.*

The doctor postponed her chemotherapy since her family had planned a vacation in Maui at the time of her diagnosis. She didn't feel sick, so she had no trouble pretending for two weeks that she didn't have cancer. They kayaked and snorkeled in the iridescent waters that lapped the sandy beaches. Cool breezes tousled their hair as they zip-lined over the Kapalua Mountains.

Perched on the peak of the Haleakala Volcano, they gazed at the sun as it wakened the dawn. The fiery globe rose as if from the blackened waters of the sea. As light splashed blazing orange rays across the sky, they mounted their bikes and cycled down the path to the volcano's base. Not once did she think about cancer. Besides, she didn't have cancer.

Upon her return from Maui, the surgeon placed an implantable IV port under the skin in her chest. The nurses infused chemotherapy agents through this port once every three weeks for six treatments. Her husband offered to stay with her during chemotherapy, but she refused. His presence during treatment threatened to shatter her illusion. *I am not getting chemotherapy. I don't have cancer.*

He would drop her off in the morning and pick her up after work. Thankfully, the drugs lulled her to sleep, despite her uncomfortable position. She was forced to sit more upright than she preferred, since her IV pump alarmed if she reclined.

IN HER SHOES: DANCING IN THE SHADOW OF CANCER

The first week after chemotherapy, Sue met her personal trainer at the gym for her regular workouts. She wasn't sick, and she wouldn't allow herself to get sick. Prior to her arrival, he sanitized all of the equipment, minimizing her risk for infection.

By the second week, her blood counts dropped too low to work out at the gym, so she ran on her home treadmill. Fatigued by the third week, she flopped onto the couch after her workouts and bonded with Judge Judy, her new daytime companion. If she attempted to rise, waves of nausea swept over her like a churning sea. The laundry would have to wait. She was grateful her girls had just left for college, leaving her with few responsibilities. With each cycle of chemotherapy, the fatigue and nausea grew progressively worse.

Only in prayer did she acknowledge the cancer. *God, please make this go away!* Sue felt confident that God would heal her. Death was not an option.

Despite her decreasing activity level, Sue discovered that one of her chemotherapy agents was a successful treatment for rheumatoid arthritis. Her arthritis went into remission. She no longer required medication.

> Yet I am confident I will see the LORD's goodness while I am here
> in the land of the living. (Psalm 27:13 NLT)

Prayer: Thank you, Lord, for allowing me the luxury of denial as a way to cope with cancer.

Chapter 56

FREEDOM!

Sue had never sported a great curly mane. Her reflection in the mirror betrayed short, limp hair of unknown natural color. If her hair fell out due to chemotherapy, she would be okay. At least chemotherapy could grant her two wishes—curly hair and weight loss.

The wig specialist provided her with her first chemotherapy lesson. She told her that hair loss usually begins two weeks after the first treatment. They pulled and tugged wigs over her head, matching Sue's current hair color and style. But the mirror reflected an image of a woman twenty years older. With her sister's help, she chose a totally different look—a blonder, short bob with bangs. The youthful Sue generated many compliments.

As predicted, two weeks after her first chemotherapy treatment, wisps of hair clung to brushes and bedding. Clumps circled the shower drain. She shuddered at the thought of being stared at in public due to bare patches on her head resembling some gross scalp disease. The time had come to shave her head.

Despite Sue's assurances that she was fine, her sister insisted on accompanying her to the salon. Her sister also planned to purchase a scarf for her, chauffeur her to chemotherapy, and postpone any consulting jobs until Sue recovered. Except for the hairdresser's appointment, Sue nixed her sister's agenda completely.

"Please shave this off," she begged as she hopped into the chair.

The hairdresser used a razor to buzz Sue's scalp, clipping the last of her tendrils.

Freedom! She swung around and caught sight of her sister. Trembling lips and pallor divulged her sister's misgivings, qualms she didn't share.

Later, when hot flashes erupted like spewing volcanoes, Sue's bald head proved advantageous. Without hair to fuss over, baldness was a major timesaver. She grabbed a scarf to dash to the mailbox or shook out her wig for special occasions.

After chemotherapy, Sue expected curly hair, but she didn't anticipate a black and white afro. A coal black patch emerged from the nape of her neck. Black tufts sprouted through the woolly white coat and created a speckled pattern. Neither shade reflected her natural color. Until hair dye could be applied, Sue's wig hid her spotted mop.

Chemotherapy granted one of her wishes, curly hair. As for Sue's other wish, her weight remained unchanged.

> Your beauty should not come from outward adornment, such as elaborate hairstyles and the wearing of gold jewelry or fine clothes. Rather, it should be that of your inner self, the unfading beauty of a gentle and quiet spirit, which is of great worth in God's sight. (1 Peter 3:3-4 NIV)

Prayer: Lord, you opened my eyes to see new possibilities in difficult situations. Thank you for the freedom and acceptance I found even in circumstances not of my choosing.

Chapter 57

HELPFUL HINTS: CARE OF THE BALD HEAD

1. Use a mild shampoo on your bald head, followed by a drop of conditioner to moisturize your scalp.

2. Wear a hat in the sun.

3. Stretchy cloth swim caps are available at swim shops for swimming and other outdoor water activities. These caps also provide a covering for the bald head and maintain warmth in an indoor pool.

4. Sleep caps help to keep your head warm at night.

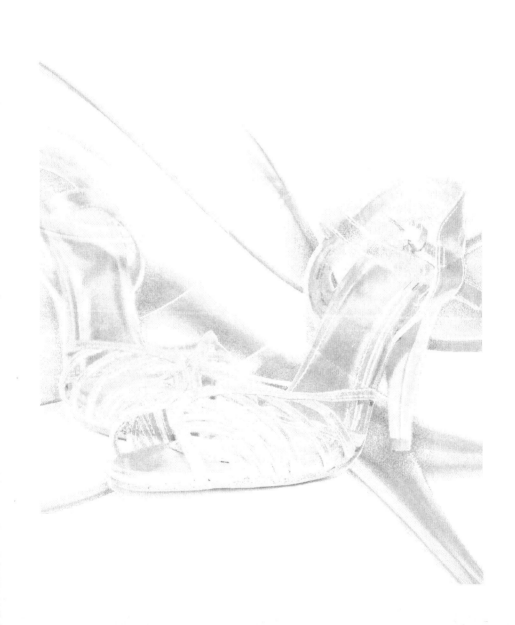

Chapter 58

SNAFU

Trudging up and down basement stairs, Sue lugged boxes of trash and treasure to the dumpster. Sweat beaded on her forehead and mingled with the dusty residue. Once again, she rolled up her sleeves and pitched in to help her friend unload her husband's hoarded books and papers.

Exhausted but satisfied, she arrived home and discovered a message from her oncologist on the answering machine. That morning she had endured another chest CT, her follow-up for non-Hodgkin's lymphoma.

"Your CT scan shows that three inches of tubing from the IV port in your chest has broken off and wedged in your heart," the doctor said. "Since your last CT was three months ago, we don't know when it broke. I notified a heart surgeon to retrieve the fragment. In the meantime, avoid heavy lifting."

Sue clutched her chest, her heart pounding. *Great! I've spent my day lifting heavy boxes, and I'm leaving for Europe in ten days.* Her oldest daughter was studying in Rome for three weeks. She planned to join her and travel throughout Europe.

Six days before her vacation, she lay on a cold, steel table, sedated in a twilight state. As the doctor poked the surgical instrument through her groin, she winced. He snaked the apparatus through her blood vessels, weaving the probe to her heart. Like an angler proud of his catch, he snagged the broken fragment but refused to remove the rest of the IV port. The doctor who'd placed the port was responsible for removal, but he was unavailable before Sue's departure to Europe.

"I don't want to leave the country with this broken port still in my chest," Sue confided to her recovery room nurse. "What if another piece breaks off?"

Late that evening, the nurse stepped away from Sue's bedside. Upon her return, she announced that she had located the doctor's partner. He agreed to remove the port at eight o'clock the next morning.

With a sigh of relief, Sue sank into the bed, grateful for her resourceful nurse.

She arrived at the doctor's office the following morning. After glancing at the doctor's calendar, the receptionist informed her that he wouldn't arrive until nine o'clock, and she wasn't scheduled.

Undaunted, Sue waited.

As he promised, the doctor arrived, injected a local anesthetic, and removed the port embedded beneath her skin. While his hands deftly manipulated the instruments, he expounded upon Europe's historic sights and architectural magnificence.

Sue had sailed over another hurdle. Next stop, Rome.

> It was the LORD our God himself who ... protected us on our entire journey and among all the nations through which we traveled. (Joshua 24:17 NIV)

Prayer: Lord, there are times I have no idea that anything is wrong. But you know. In my ignorance, I sometimes place myself at risk for harm. Thank you for protecting me.

Part 6

Rita: Breast Cancer

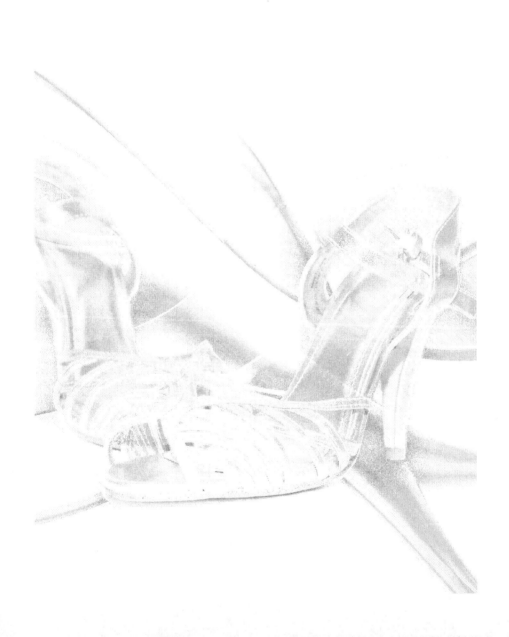

Chapter 59

Are There Phones in Heaven?

Under the cover of darkness, Rita slipped out the back door and sank onto the creaky wooden swing. Despite the warm evening, a shiver raced down her spine. The events of the past few weeks clamored for her attention and competed with the incessant chirping of the crickets. Precious thoughts of her husband and three sons swirled around her mind, memories threatened to be swept away by cancer.

At age thirty-nine, Rita had discovered a lump in her left breast while weaning her third son. Busy juggling a family and a teaching career in special education, she dismissed the lump as a clogged milk duct. But as the weeks passed, the lump refused to dissolve.

An ultrasound revealed a couple suspicious nodules hanging onto scar tissue from a benign fibroid removed when she was eighteen. Despite the doctor's warning of a 90% chance of cancer, Rita never heard the "C" word. She clung to the echo of the doctor's voice. *There's a ten percent chance the lump is benign.* Rita and her husband decided not to tell their older boys, ages eleven and eight, until they were sure of her diagnosis.

Under the distant glow of stars and the occasional flicker of fireflies, Rita prayed as the swing rhythmically swayed. If only this rocking motion could lull her into a peaceful sleep and calm her fears like rocking had soothed her babies.

The back door slammed and roused Rita from the cacophony of the night. Springing down the steps and across the lawn, her eight-year-old son with autism plopped next to her on the swing. Bunching his white T-shirt, he nuzzled against her left side near the lump. Rita draped her arm around his slender shoulders. As her cheek brushed his tousled hair, a whiff of little boy sweat wafted toward her nostrils. His blue jean clad legs dangled over the wooden slats while mother and son rocked in the swing.

With a smudged, upturned face, her son stared into the heavens. "Mom, I've been thinking a lot lately … do you think Jesus has phones in heaven? Because if I die before you, I'd like to call you. Do you think Jesus has phones in heaven?"

Rita drew in a sharp breath, her heart pierced. *Does he know more than we think?* "I believe Jesus has phones in heaven," Rita replied. "I'll make you a deal. If I go to heaven before you, I'll ask Jesus if I can call you."

"Oh, good!" Her son hopped off the swing, bounded across the yard, and jumped onto a large boulder. With outstretched arms, he took his stand. "Mom, do you think Walt Disney is making movies in heaven?"

"I think he is making his best movies in heaven."

"Me too, Mom!"

Rita smiled through the tears glistening in her eyes. She hoped and prayed that her son would not be robbed of a childhood that revolved around his mom and the wonderful world of Disney.

> For great is your love, higher than the heavens; your faithfulness reaches to the skies. (Psalm 108:4 NIV)

Prayer: Lord, as I gaze into the heavens, each star hung in place, I'm reminded of how great your love is toward me. Thank you, Lord, for your amazing love and care for me.

Chapter 60

CHIP AWAY

Beneath glaring lights, Rita gripped the edge of the exam table while the doctors inserted a needle into her left breast without anesthesia. Three times they huddled over her as they jabbed and withdrew the needle then scurried to the lab with each specimen. She noted a slower pace each time they returned. Her teacher intuition kicked in. *This doesn't look very good.*

"You are very brave woman," the Egyptian doctor said, resting his gloved hand upon her arm.

Rita didn't feel very brave. The force of her circumstances had propelled her into this exam room, not courage.

Perched on her husband's lap, her twenty-two-month-old son kept a watchful eye on his mom. Despite reassurances to the contrary, she worried her baby would be traumatized by the day's events. Her fears culminated that evening when he squirmed in her arms, shook his head, and refused to nurse from her left breast. Rita's heart sank. *Even my baby knows something's wrong.*

The next week, doctors removed six more tumor samples during a core biopsy. At least she received a local anesthetic and had the privilege of watching the procedure on a black and white television screen. There certainly couldn't be any cancer left.

Yet, two days after Thanksgiving, Rita once again lay on a cold exam table while the doctor injected blue dye into the tumor site. "This doesn't hurt very much," the doctor said.

She squeezed the technician's hand and grimaced. The dye stung. A lot. The dye targeted the lymph node nearest the cancer. The node would be biopsied during her lumpectomy later that day.

After the biopsy and lumpectomy, Rita curled her arm around her stomach and willed the churning to stop. The nausea from anesthesia competed with the sickening news. The doctors had found cancer in the lymph node and suspected the disease had spread. Rita just wanted to go home. The nurses whisked her, slumped over in her wheel chair and vomiting, out to the car.

That evening, one of Rita's former students with autism arrived on her doorstep along with his mother. His beaming face peeked around two brown bags of groceries nestled in his arms. He had picked out his favorite super foods to keep Rita healthy and insisted upon paying for them with his own money.

Though quivering and weak, Rita smiled as she leaned against the doorframe, touched by his kindness and generosity. He couldn't afford these groceries. After he deposited the bags on the counter, she stretched out her arms, offering a hug.

"Everyone wants to hug me today," he said with a sheepish grin.

Little by little, the biopsies chiseled away at the tumor. A phone call she received at school dealt the final blow. Not all of the cancer had been removed.

"I can't handle any more of these little biopsies. Let's just do the mastectomy."

> Be strong and courageous. Do not be afraid; do not be discouraged, for the Lord your God will be with you wherever you go. (Joshua 1:9 NIV)

Prayer: Lord, sometimes I don't feel very brave. Thank you for giving me the courage to walk through the hard places.

Chapter 61

ALLELUIA

Behind closed doors, Rita perched on a vinyl chair during her pre-operative consultation with the nurse.

"Alleluia! Alleluia!" Rita heard her two-year-old son sing out through the door. Grandma was pushing him in his stroller through the hallways as she waited for Rita's consultation to end, and Rita knew her mom was praying for the best outcome for her daughter, all while the boy belted out the Celtic Alleluia sung in church every Sunday.

The surgeon laid out the details for Rita's upcoming mastectomy as well as her options for reconstruction. But one thing she knew for certain—she wanted her mastectomy, chemotherapy port, and reconstruction all done in one surgery. Anesthesia made her sick.

With surgery still two days away, she asked, "Is it possible for the plastic surgeon to do my reconstruction at the same time?"

"He wouldn't be available on such short notice," the nurse replied.

"It couldn't hurt to call him," Rita suggested.

The nurse hesitated, and then reluctantly agreed.

When she returned, the nurse exclaimed, "He actually answered his phone. He never does!" Her eyes widened in amazement. "He'll be right down."

In the meantime, Rita's mom rolled in with her little cherub.

The plastic surgeon arrived and listened to Rita's request for an all-in-one surgery. He stroked his chin, checked his schedule, and briefly examined her. "Oh, yes, this is very doable." He turned toward Rita's mom. "We'll take good care of her," he reassured her.

God had answered Grandma's prayer, punctuated by the praises of her grandson. Alleluia!

From the lips of children and infants you, Lord, have called forth your praise. (Matthew 21:16 NIV)

Prayer: Thank you, Lord, for reminding me that you hear our prayers and delight in the praises of your children.

Chapter 62

RECONSTRUCTED TO WHOLENESS

"Who did your reconstruction?" the radiology tech asked Rita during her follow-up mammogram for breast cancer. "I've never seen such good work."

Rita smiled as she recalled the stages of her reconstruction. The first stage had occurred during her mastectomy. While the oncology surgeon removed her left breast and lymph nodes, the plastic surgeon started on her abdomen, removing her C-section scars along with her naval. He tunneled part of her abdominal muscle and fat across her chest, now minus a breast, and attached the tissue beneath her collarbone. Her pregnancy stretch marks splayed across her newly mounted breast, a tribute to her three sons. As a finishing touch, he embroidered her naval back into the rightful place. In the past, one woman had sued when they had forgotten to replace her belly button.

Early the following morning, the surgeon greeted Rita, who was still groggy from anesthesia. The doctor's lab coat hung open, revealing the string of pearls that always encircled her neck. Even in the dim light, the three diamond rings on her left hand sparkled as she examined Rita.

Smiling, the doctor said, "Everything looks good."

A short time later, the intern arrived. Rita slipped her glasses over her nose.

"What's with the glasses?" he asked, noticing the safety pins slid between the bows and the frame.

"I have three boys," Rita replied.

"Oh, I see." The intern threw back his head and laughed. He examined the black and blue baseball, complete with sutures, mounted on Rita's chest. "I did most of your plastic surgery—under supervision, of course," he boasted.

When the swelling had decreased and the bruises faded, her plastic surgeon nodded his head and rocked back on his heels. "That's my best work," he said with a smug grin plastered between his puffed cheeks. "I would like to photograph the stages of your reconstruction for my medical journals."

Rita drew back and paused. "I guess that would be okay." Besides, the mound on her chest didn't feel like her but felt more like a cold, numb, separate entity. She didn't care who saw photos of her reconstructed breast. *He might as well snap pictures of my bare arm.*

Several months after surgery, the doctor twisted and pulled tight a small amount of tissue in the center of her new breast and formed a bud, thereby creating a nipple. After healing had taken place, the nurse tattooed around the bud with tiny needles, matching the natural shade of her areola. Still numb, Rita experienced minimal pain during these procedures.

With her reconstruction complete, she felt like the surgical mound on her chest had finally morphed into her own body. She was whole.

> For He bruises, but He binds up; He wounds, but His hands make whole. (Job 5:18 NKJV)

Prayer: Thank you, Lord, that when I'm bruised and wounded, you heal me and make me whole, even though sometimes my wholeness may look different than I would have liked.

Chapter 63

THE EMOTIONAL PLUNGE

Steroids coursed through Rita's veins. Her heart raced and every muscle fiber tingled. She had survived her first round of chemotherapy, despite the defibrillator paddles parked next to her bed.

As she headed home, a burst of energy spurred her on to clean out her closet. Sort. Pitch. Organize.

But upon her arrival home, fatigue sapped her strength. Her shoulders sagged. The invitation to slump in an overstuffed chair trumped the enticement to clean her bulging closets. Maybe tomorrow.

The next day, Rita's emotions plunged into a churning black quagmire of depression. Why'd she get married and have these kids? Her gaze lingered on the furnishings and the knick-knacks scattered about the room. Why'd she buy all this stuff? Her nerve endings tingled as if spidery legs scurried beneath her skin. She had to get out of this body. Her skin crawled. She clutched her head between her trembling hands. *I'm going crazy!*

Humor helped to keep her sane and distracted her from the jitters. As she lounged on the couch with her family, their laughter echoed throughout the room as they watched funny movies and reruns of *I Love Lucy*. But even between the slapstick comedies, mortality lurked in the recesses of her mind. She'd probably never see this movie again.

Rita lashed out at her husband. "As soon as I die, there will be someone waiting in the wings for you to marry!" she fumed. "She won't even care about my boys." Worry over who would take care of her sons consumed her days and nights, robbing her of sleep. "Besides, why should that other woman get all my jewelry?"

Her husband had always stood by her, but this time he stood with his hands in his pockets, silenced by his wife's accusations.

Mortified by her ranting, Rita sank deeper into despondency.

Much dialogue ensued between her and her husband regarding their will. In the end, they tabled their discussion without resolution. When they purchased a double cemetery plot, Rita's spirits lifted. "At least if I die first, we'll be buried together," she said. "That other woman probably won't want you to be buried with me."

After her last chemotherapy treatment, her husband cooked her favorite meal—steak. They celebrated her victory with a bottle of sparkling grape juice.

"You've been so strong through everything," Rita said to her husband. "I never saw you cry."

"I didn't want you to see me cry," he said. "I was afraid of how it would affect you emotionally."

"It would've been okay," she reassured him, now that her emotions had stabilized.

"But you didn't need that," he said. "You needed me to be strong."

He was right. Rita needed him to be her anchor.

Cast all your anxiety on him because he cares for you. (1 Peter 5:7 NIV)

Prayer: Lord, please help me to cope with my emotions and not lash out when I feel as though I'm falling to pieces. Remind me to bring all my anxious thoughts to you because you love me.

Chapter 64

A DREAM FULFILLED

Rita hauled herself out of bed, stumbled to the window, and parted the curtains. In the middle of her chemotherapy cycle, she had registered to attend a women's day-away conference, featuring vocalist Kathy Troccoli as the keynote speaker. She'd always admired Kathy's rich alto voice.

Staring through the pane, she breathed a prayer, "Lord, if it be your will, let me have an opportunity to say hello to Kathy today."

Arriving alone, Rita braved a crowd of twelve hundred women with a red scarf wrapped around her bald head.

A nearby voice announced, "There's Kathy Troccoli!"

The woman next to her briefly vacated her seat.

Rita turned her head in the designated direction.

Kathy locked eyes with Rita. Leaving the soundboard, she approached Rita and sat down. "Are you going through chemo?" Kathy asked.

With her red scarf draping her shoulder, Rita nodded.

"My mom went through chemo," Kathy said. "I remember combing her long black hair. It was so hard watching strands fall out in my hands. You're very brave to be going through chemo."

During the course of their conversation, Rita shared her concerns for her three young sons. Kathy prayed for her that she would live throughout her motherhood.

During the keynote address, Rita devoured the nuggets of faith that Kathy shared from her heart. After lunch, nausea forced her to leave the conference before Kathy's concert.

But Kathy autographed her CD and thrust several of her books into her hands. "When I come back, I want you to show me your hair."

Shortly after the conference, Rita sat in her oncologist's office.

"How long do you think you'll live?" he asked.

"Throughout my motherhood," she replied, echoing Kathy's prayer. This prayer had now become a lifeline for Rita when assailed with fears, doubts, and questions.

"How long is that?"

"I plan to see my children's children," she replied.

A grin spread across his face. He never asked her that question again.

Kathy didn't return to Rita's hometown, but when Rita's hair reappeared, she left a message on Kathy's website: *My blonde hair has grown back—the woman in the red scarf.*

Rita treasured those precious moments with Kathy. She discovered that sometimes when we ask for little things, God gives so much more than we can imagine.

> Now to him who is able to do immeasurably more than all we ask
> or imagine ... to him be glory. (Ephesians 3:20-21 NIV)

Prayer: Thank you, Lord, for reminding me that you care about the little things that are important to me, and you delight in answering my prayers with wonderful surprises.

Chapter 65

THE SQUEEZE

"Are you going through chemotherapy?" an elderly couple asked Rita one Sunday, noting the colorful scarf that draped her bald head. "Our daughter never missed a day of work during her chemo," they bragged as they leaned over the scratched wooden pew.

Once again, the guilt of not working piled up like waste in a sewage plant. Well-meaning friends spewed remarks such as "I know people who never took off work. They didn't have benefits." The guilt parade continued. She was grateful she carried long-term disability insurance through the school district.

Since each chemotherapy treatment escalated her level of fatigue, her doctors advocated for a fourteen-month leave of absence. But her doctor's restrictions proved to be no match for the disability insurance carrier. The insurance company demanded their money back, requiring her to apply for another form of disability that offered a lesser amount of money.

The benefits personnel phoned Rita to inform her they were sending forms for her to sign.

"Why are you calling me?" she asked.

"Well, I'm explaining to you why you have to sign this form," she said. "This isn't that hard to understand," the woman chided.

"Just send me the paperwork so I can read it!" Rita said, frustrated and feeling like a chastised child. Even in her debilitated state, she knew she had a right to review all legal forms.

Besides the paperwork, the insurance company hired a woman to question her regarding her daily activities. She demanded that Rita account for every hour of every day and hounded her with questions. What do you do in the morning, the afternoon, evening, weekends? How often?

Being a detailed-oriented person and struggling with chemotherapy's brain fog, the interrogation proved especially grueling.

The insurance carrier forced her to appear in court. Clad in a dark business suit, the lawyer opened a large, hard-cover book with worn edges. Flipping to the designated page in the constitutional manual, he locked his steely eyes with the judge and said, "She is a special education teacher." With his finger, he found his place in the manual, "This activity is considered moderately sedentary with moderate mental and physical activity …"

"Excuse me," Rita interjected, "but did you talk to my supervisor and principal to find out what I really do?'

"I don't need to," he replied. "This is what the book says."

"I'm not the average special education teacher," Rita countered. "I teach autistic kids. I do a lot of physical lifting as well as care for disabled children on tube feedings." Rita felt her cheeks flush with anger. "I have a very high energy job and rarely sit down at my desk. I can't even complete my computer work until after school."

In the courtroom, they continued to discuss Rita, excluding her from the conversation.

She felt invisible. During her testimony, her dangling earrings quivered beneath her turban wrapped scarf. Sobs racked her shoulders as she hunched over in her chair, caged by its rungs.

With a hardness that matched his judicial bench, the judge stopped the proceedings. "Let's give her a few minutes to pull herself together." A lack of compassion emanated throughout the courtroom.

In the end, the disability insurance company won. They recovered their money.

> I know that the LORD secures justice for the poor and upholds the cause of the needy. (Psalm 140:12 NIV)

Prayer: Lord, I don't understand why you allow me to go through such humiliation and loss of finances, but you know what it feels like to be wrongly accused and humiliated. I trust you to take care of me despite my circumstances.

Chapter 66

Flipped Wigs

Rita and several friends gathered at an Asian restaurant for lunch, a refuge from the blustery winds.

"My daughter was mortified," Rita's friend confided in hushed tones as their chopsticks clicked. Tears welled up in her eyes and threatened to trickle into her lo mein noodles.

Earlier that day, as Rita's friend strode across the library parking lot toting a stack of books, a swirling gust of wind whisked the wig off her bald head. As the hairpiece tumbled across the pavement, she yelled at her daughter, "Hurry up and get it!"

With a stomp of her foot, her daughter trapped the renegade wig. She grasped the unruly hairpiece and plopped it on her mom's bald head. "Put your books on top of your head," the daughter said, exasperated. "After all, you have those library books for a reason." She tromped ahead without a backward glance.

Another woman chimed in. That morning, she purchased a mirror for her college-bound daughter. As she lugged the bulky package to the car, a blast of air hijacked her wig and flung it across the parking lot, tossing it like a scrap of paper past trucks and SUVs.

Her daughter chased the elusive wig and landed the tresses with her shoe. "My daughter was so embarrassed," she said. Just like her friend, tears glistened in her eyes.

Rita had dodged the flying wig escapades. Instead of wigs, she donned brightly colored scarves and dangling earrings. As she imagined these scenarios, the corners of her mouth curled in amusement. The humiliating tears of her friends compelled her to choke back the laughter that bubbled beneath her reconstructed breast. She tried to feel compassion. But how ironic to shed tears over flipped wigs while one battles for life.

> You are those who have stood by me in my trials. (Luke 22:28 NIV)

Prayer: Thank you Lord, for the friends who share in my struggles and stand by me when I feel embarrassed. Help me to be compassionate and understanding of others in their humiliating trials.

Chapter 67

Through the Eyes of a Child

"Remember, Rita, make sure you tell your children what's happening—not necessarily the specifics, but children know when something's wrong," Rita's friend who worked at the hospice center counseled her. "Ask them why they think you got cancer."

One night after Rita's two older sons climbed into their bunks, Rita asked the gnawing question, "Why do you think Mommy got cancer?"

Her eleven-year-old son dropped his gaze. "Because I drank from you?" he mumbled.

Rita's heart ached, recognizing the guilt that resonated in her son's voice. "Oh, no, honey, you helped Mommy to live longer." As she hugged him, he buried his head in her chest. His stiffened shoulders sagged, hopefully released from the weight of guilt.

Every night at bedtime, Rita blessed and prayed for each of her sons as she tucked them into bed. "Lord, help my boys to sleep well and wake up ready to serve you in the day to come. In Jesus's name we pray. Amen, amen, amen."

One night, her middle son popped out from under his covers and said, "Mom, can I pray for you?"

"That would be great, "Rita said.

He extended his arm and rested his little palm on her bald head. "Dear Jesus, please help my mom be healthy and strong and grow her hair back. In your name we pray. Amen, amen, and amen."

Rita hugged her son and thanked him for his beautiful prayer. She worried that somehow in his mind, she wouldn't be all right until her hair grew back, especially since he had protested and cried when she shaved her head.

Every night thereafter, he raced into the living room, "Mom, Mom, I forgot to pray for you!"

"Each day I'm here with you," she reassured him, "I'm okay."

Her eleven-year-old son celebrated the end of Mom's chemo with a drawing—a sad-faced green blob of cancer devoured by a razor-toothed chemo shark. Not to be outdone, her eight-year-old drew a chemo mousetrap with a balloon floating at its edge. When popped, the balloon killed the cancer. She presented copies of these pictures to her oncologist who hung them in his office along with his own children's artwork.

Rita completed her chemo. Once again, thick blonde hair cascaded over her shoulders. In the eyes of her sons, Mom was well.

> But Jesus said, "Let the children come to me. Don't stop them!
> For the Kingdom of Heaven belongs to those who are like these
> children." (Matthew 19:14 NLT)

Prayer: Thank you, Lord, that you not only take care of me when I'm sick, but you care about my children too.

Chapter 68

FACING MORTALITY

"Rita, how do you feel about facing your mortality?" A young teacher asked while they packed up after class.

"What do you mean?" Rita replied.

"Well, your chances of dying are much higher than someone who doesn't have cancer," he reasoned.

"You know what, you could go outside today and get hit by a car," she said. "Just because I'm sick doesn't mean I'm going to die before other people."

At first, the bluntness of these questions astounded her. But as time marched on, she realized her cancer diagnosis served as a springboard for many conversations about God and mortality, even among the non-religious.

Since she taught some challenging special education students, she appreciated the adeptness of her Irish teaching assistant. Occasionally, she'd overhear her chide one of the students in her Irish brogue, "I hate to burst your bubble, but Miss Rita loves all of her students the same. You are no better than anyone else."

Rita forged a special bond with this aide.

"Oh, Rita, I would love to take you to Ireland and visit those places that no one else will show you."

Her sweet cadence reminded her of her own Irish heritage.

One day after class the aide said, "My dear Rita, I'm so sorry you had to go through cancer. It's just not fair."

"None of us know when we'll go," Rita replied. "It's okay. My cancer treatment is behind me. I'll be here as long as the Lord wants me here."

At the close of the school year, her teaching assistant gave her a parting hug and said, "We'll get together this summer after we get back from our trip."

Two days later while on vacation, her beloved Irish teaching assistant died in a car accident—a tragedy that reminded her that all of her days are in God's hands.

On another occasion, she visited a friend dying from lung cancer in the hospice center. Memories of other women who'd passed on lingered in her mind. *They were all doing better than I.* Rita sat close by her friend and rubbed her slim shoulder, the only comfort she could offer to one in such great pain. But she felt targeted by the dying woman's angry tears mingled with tears of sadness.

Rita had the audacity to live. *Why am I still here? She has children too.* The tentacles of survivor guilt latched onto her heart.

My kids still need me. Am I going to be next? Worried that she would become a stranger to her boys prompted Rita to videotape herself and share the precious memories she carried. She refused to be forgotten.

> Your eyes saw my unformed body; all the days ordained for me were written in your book before one of them came to be. (Psalm 139:16 NIV)

Prayer: Thank you, Lord, that the days of my life are in your hands. Help me to rest in your peace when I'm afraid of what the future will bring.

Chapter 69

REPERCUSSIONS

Rita tugged the sleep cap over her shiny scalp. No sooner had she tucked the blankets under her chin than a blast of heat radiated from beneath her skin. Sweat plastered her gown to her chest. She whipped off her cap and covers. The frigid air laced the dampness clinging to her emerging goose bumps. Huddled under her covers once again, she braced herself for the next flash.

Her chemotherapy had hurled her into early menopause.

Despite remission, the aftermath of chemotherapy's demolition persisted. A befuddling fog had settled over her brain. In mid-sentence, her mouth gaped. The words that wrapped around her tongue dissolved before being verbalized. The alphabet cued her to names but failed to aid her spelling or illegible handwriting. Lists and notes littered her desk at school and her refrigerator at home. Her memory had short-circuited. Chemo brain clouded her thinking, affected her ability to concentrate, focus, organize, and multi-task. Even after chemotherapy, the fog persisted.

Rita cried out in pain as charley horses raced up and down the front and back of her legs in opposite directions. While her husband stretched one side, she countered with the other. Sit-ups, bending, and rotating prodded the charley horses to gallop through the reconstruction in her chest. At least swimming and biking provided some relief.

The removal of twelve lymph nodes during cancer surgery interrupted the flow of lymphatic fluid and resulted in swelling along the arm on the side of her mastectomy—lymphedema. The doctors recommended she wear a compression sleeve, but an internet search revealed a manual drainage technique. While her husband massaged down her neck, back, and arm, the fluid shifted. The arm movement involved with knitting also helped to control the swelling. Permanent restrictions resulted from the lymphedema—no heavy lifting, no IVs, blood draws, or blood pressures in that arm.

Cancer also crimped her exercise routine. Would she ever be able to run again? Just walking winded her. With a shortened and stiff Achilles tendon, she pushed herself forward as she plodded uphill then downhill. *I'm so tired.* Push. Push. *Another five minutes.* Without a fight, her muscles would cripple with contractions.

Rita trudged one mile in the Race for the Cure, determined to meet the challenge. Eventually she fought her way back to running sprints.

As with any cancer, recurrence hovers in the recesses of Rita's mind like a polluting haze. Despite her mastectomy, reconstruction, chemotherapy, and the lingering side effects, Rita remains grateful that she is able to raise her sons. She also enjoys teaching, running, gardening and knitting prayer scarves.

> I have fought the good fight, I have finished the race, and I have remained faithful. (2 Timothy 4:7 NLT)

Prayer: Sometimes life doesn't turn out as I hoped or planned. But I thank you, Lord, that nothing interferes with your plans and purposes for my life. You will bring good out of all that has happened to me.

Part 7

Ruth: Ovarian Cancer

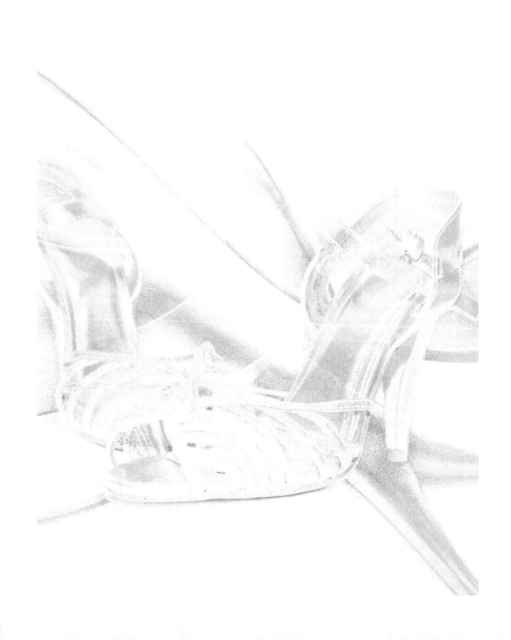

Chapter 70

WILL SOMEONE LISTEN?

Ruth brushed her hand over the tender nodule that had surfaced along the inner aspect of her upper arm. Hot and purple-red. As a nurse, she diagnosed herself with a blood clot.

Since her family doctor was unavailable, she scheduled an appointment with his colleague. The doctor insisted that the pain and swelling in Ruth's arm were related to an injury.

"But I didn't injure my arm," Ruth said. "The spot looks like a blood clot to me."

Minimizing Ruth's concerns, the doctor ordered an antibiotic. She noted that Ruth's uterus resisted normal mobility on her pelvic exam, so she ordered an ultrasound of the abdomen and pelvis.

"I'll see you back here in six months," the doctor said.

After the ultrasound, Ruth phoned the clinic several times for her results, but no one returned her calls.

Two weeks after the lump appeared on her arm, Ruth noticed raised purple-red spots on the top of her foot. Once again Ruth's nursing instinct kicked in—phlebitis. The swollen and painful foot protested at her attempts to wiggle into a shoe.

She returned to the same doctor who now ordered Ruth to elevate her foot and stay off work for a few days.

"I've never had these symptoms before," Ruth said. "Shouldn't we be digging a little deeper?"

The doctor ordered several blood tests. She later prescribed iron pills for Ruth but never explored the cause of the anemia.

In the meantime, Ruth waited for the usual postcard stamped with normal test results. The card never arrived. Multiple times she phoned the clinic to obtain her lab results, but once again, they neglected to return her calls.

One Sunday morning, pain surged through her hip joint. Barely able to flex her hip, she limped across the room, grasping at nearby furniture. Something was terribly wrong.

She phoned the clinic Monday morning to schedule a visit with their family doctor, instead of the doctor she'd been seeing. Since the family doctor would also be delivering babies, they couldn't give her a specific appointment time and placed her on the wait list.

In the clinic waiting room, Ruth lowered herself into a hardback chair. She wished her husband could be with her, but he needed to tend their dairy farm. Between glances at the clock, she rubbed her hip and shifted in her seat, attempting to soothe the persistent throb. Minutes ticked into hours as she waited.

The doctor strolled into the exam room five hours later. *Now someone will listen.* As he flipped open her chart, a sheaf of papers tumbled out. Five weeks of her never-mailed test results lay strewn across the linoleum floor. He bent down and gathered the slips of paper, shuffling through the results. Silently, he turned away and peered out the window. He was not only their family doctor, but also a friend. He'd attended college with her husband.

Slowly, he turned back to face Ruth. "I'm sorry you had to be postponed and not dealt with in the proper way." He paused, pursing his lips. "I suspect you have ovarian cancer. We need to schedule a CT scan of your abdomen and pelvis. The ultrasound didn't visualize your ovaries. They either didn't find them or weren't looking for them."

Ruth stared at him in disbelief.

"I'm also concerned about the bleeding in your kidneys, so we'll schedule an intravenous pyelogram," he continued. "We need to do some blood tests including a CA 125, the ovarian cancer marker."

She collapsed in her chair, too choked up to speak. Her shoulders convulsed as she sobbed.

Two days later, she arrived at the hospital at eight o'clock a.m. for her CT scan. Numb, she followed their instructions, still shocked from her presumed diagnosis.

At noon, the doctor phoned her, "Can your husband bring you into the hospital right away?"

Upon admission to the hospital, they started IV heparin to treat the immediate threat—blood clots. They needed to reduce the risk of increased clot formation before surgery. The doctor arranged for her to be transferred by ambulance to a larger hospital thirty minutes away that specialized in oncology.

As the test results came in, a clearer picture of Ruth's health emerged. Within two days, the doctors confirmed her diagnosis—ovarian cancer. They surmised the tumor secreted calcium that ultimately transformed her body into a clot factory. The malignancy spit multiple blood clots throughout her legs, peppered her lungs, and showered her kidneys, which caused the bleeding. The enlarged tumor had also triggered the hip pain.

For ten days, Ruth waited for surgery, grappling with her diagnosis of a fast-growing tumor and the risk of bleeding from the heparin dripping into her veins. Waves of anxiety crashed over her and threatened to drown her in a sea of tears. Her muscles quivered. Her heart raced, squeezing her chest. If she could just breathe, breathe …

After the ten days, the doctors shut off the heparin. Twenty-four hours later, they whisked Ruth into surgery for ovarian cancer debulking. Since the tumor encroached on the wall of her bowel, she also faced a possible colostomy, which escalated her stress level. She couldn't face looking at an angry, red stoma protruding from her abdomen for the rest of her life. The thought of the colostomy bag leaking in public mortified her.

The surgeon discovered a rare four-inch tumor connecting her ovary to the uterus. He was confident that he had removed all of the cancer. Thankfully, Ruth dodged the threatened colostomy since the cancer hadn't invaded the colon.

If Ruth had taken the advice of the first doctor and not returned for six months, she might not have survived. Miraculously, she also escaped a deadly lung clot and a stroke.

It wasn't my time.

> For you have delivered me from death and my feet from stumbling,
> that I may walk before God in the light of life. (Psalm 56:13 NIV)

Prayer: When those who should listen to me fail to hear my concerns, I'm grateful, Lord, that you listen and watch over me.

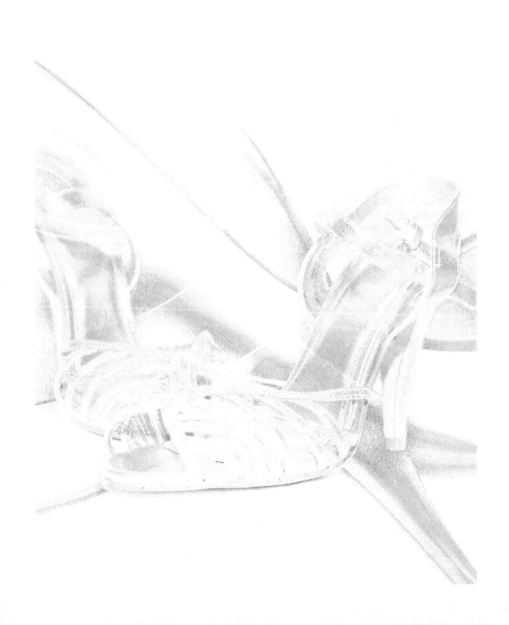

Chapter 71

Helpful Hints: Blood Clots

1. Some cancers and chemotherapy agents can increase the risk of blood clots.

2. Notify your doctor if you have the following symptoms of a blood clot: pain, redness, or swelling of an extremity, usually a calf or thigh. The extremity may appear pale or have a bluish tint. Blood clots can also occur in the arms especially on the side of an implanted venous access device.

3. Blood clots in the lungs are called pulmonary emboli and require immediate medical attention. If you experience chest pain, an irregular heartbeat, unexplained shortness of breath, or cough up blood, call 911 immediately.

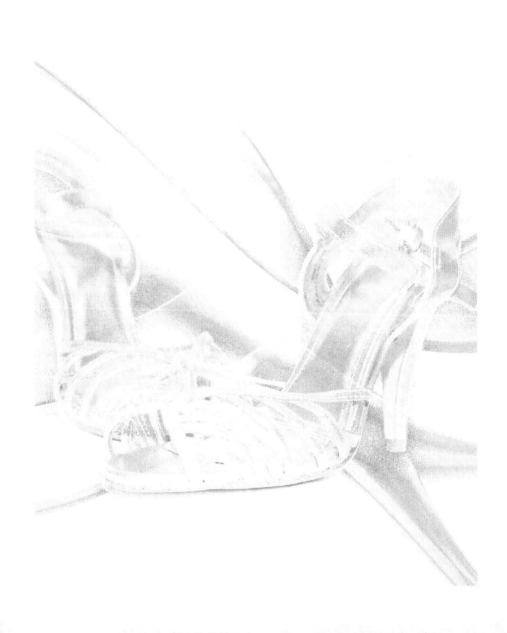

Chapter 72

SPIKED WITH TEARS

Ruth stooped over, her arm guarding her abdominal incision. Guided by the nurse's hand, she pivoted into the wheelchair. After adjusting the folds of her robe, she nodded. Her daughter accompanied her as the nurse wheeled her down the corridor of the oncology ward toward the closet at the end of the hall.

As the nurse swung open the door, she peeked into the closet. Faceless Styrofoam heads stared back. Wigs, donated by beauty salons and various women's organizations perched atop the molded forms. One by one, the nurse selected a wig, held it against Ruth's hair and attempted to match her cut and color.

Ruth chose a flattering style that met with her daughter's approval. All too soon, she would need the protective covering. The doctors planned to administer her first chemotherapy treatment before her discharge from the hospital.

Two weeks later, Ruth woke and brushed her hand across her pillow. Her fingers caught a tangled shock of hair. A sob lodged in her throat.

"I can't cope with losing my hair in clumps or shaving my head," Ruth said to her hairdresser. "I just need you to cut my hair as short as you can."

Her beautician clipped Ruth's hair to about an inch in length.

Ruth wept, her tears mingling with the thick hair discarded at her feet.

While pampering Ruth, the hairdresser sculpted her masterpiece. She squirted a dab of mousse in her palm and finger-combed it through Ruth's hair, creating a full spiked do.

As each chemotherapy cycle neared, new hair popped up, only to be snatched away by the next drug cocktail. Ruth sank to her lowest point.

She had never been a hat person. No matter what hairstyle she sported, her full-bodied hair nudged hats askew. But chemotherapy solved that problem. She purchased a few fashionable hats but settled on baseball caps for everyday wear. However, no hat warded off the chill that prickled the now-vacant nape of her neck.

One Sunday morning, she slipped on her wig for church, but as the service drew to a close, she winced. Her wig pinched along the edge of her hairline. On the way home, she whipped off the wig, exposing her bald head.

Squeals erupted from the back seat, followed by stifled giggles. "What did Grandma just do?"

Ruth glanced at her grandchildren and chuckled, joining in their merriment.

> I am worn out from my groaning. All night long I flood my bed
> with weeping and drench my couch with tears. (Psalm 6:6 NIV)

Prayer: Lord, I feel as though I've lost an integral part of who I am. I know you understand my tears and the pain of losing my hair. Thank you for the gift of laughter in the midst of the pain.

Chapter 73

Helpful Hints: Wigs

1. Make your wig-shopping day fun. Take a friend and try on different colors and styles. Go out to lunch.

2. Select a wig before chemotherapy so as to better match your hair color. Clip a swatch of hair to use later as a color reference.

3. The American Cancer Society provides free wigs.

4. The TLC catalogue is a great resource for wigs, hats, and scarves.

5. Synthetic wigs are less expensive and require minimal maintenance, compared to natural hair. Synthetic wig fibers will melt when they come in contact with steam or heat.

6. A skull cap or nylon liner help reduce the itching from wigs.

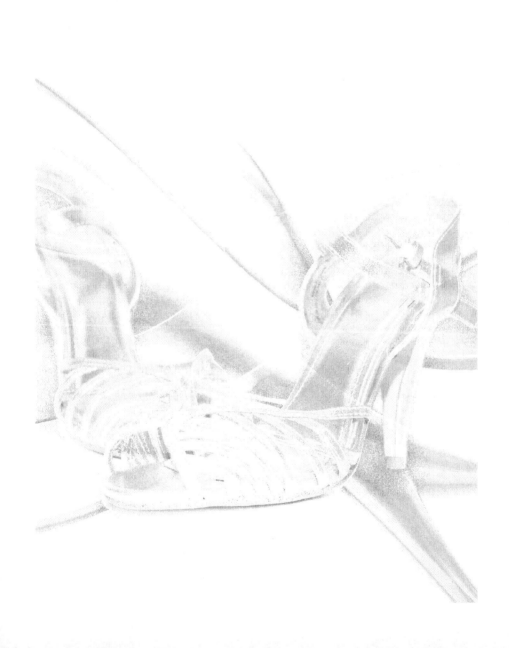

Chapter 74

WIRED AND TIRED

Ruth fidgeted beneath the tangled sheets as if a pot of espresso coursed through her veins. The real culprit proved to be the steroids that buzzed through every nerve fiber, the prelude to her morning chemotherapy. With her eyes popped open, she stared at the gray shadows flickering across the ceiling of her hospital room. Chemotherapy couldn't wait, despite her recent surgery.

The next morning after chemotherapy, Ruth's doctor discharged her from the hospital. A four-inch incision splayed open her abdomen. Three times a day, the nurses had pulled out the old gauze, donned sterile gloves, and repacked the wound. Once home, Ruth's daughter and neighbor, both nurses, managed the dressing changes. The doctor ordered her not to shower until the incision healed, so Ruth resorted to sponge baths. She remained housebound for several months until her incision closed.

What's next, Lord? she asked with mounting anxiety. Her doctor had encouraged her to return to work, but her job had become so stressful she toyed with the idea of quitting. Besides, how could she be on her feet all day and take care of her patients when she could hardly put one foot in front of the other? Her blood counts plummeted with each treatment, escalating her fatigue. Ruth declined the family leave offered by her employer. She felt her absence would place an extra burden on her co-workers, so she opted to retire.

Every four weeks for six months, she trudged into the chemotherapy clinic. Another restless night wired on steroids was followed by a day hooked up to the chemical cocktail that promised a hope-filled future. Lunch bypassed Ruth when the time rolled around at the clinic. Even though she didn't feel sick, her appetite had taken a hike with a greater marching endurance than her legs could muster. After her treatment, she leaned on her husband's arm and plodded out to the car as if invisible weights saddled her feet.

The day after chemotherapy, she dragged herself through the house. Restless energy surges betrayed her exhausted body. Sleep eluded her. Daily tasks seemed insurmountable. In a few days, the chemotherapy drugs would stoke the flu-like body aches.

Chemotherapy-induced sickness plagued Ruth that entire summer. Lethargy and low blood counts increased the risk of infection and prevented her from assisting her husband with the chores on their dairy farm. They couldn't afford to hire help, so they sold their farm and moved into town.

Even after chemotherapy ended, the demolition persisted. Arthritis had nagged at her joints before chemotherapy, but the drugs that fought the cancer also damaged her joints, resulting in unresolved pain and swelling in her feet and toes.

Cancer and chemotherapy transformed Ruth's home, her livelihood— her life. But in the end, the changes brought a new life filled with joy.

> Lord, don't hold back your tender mercies from me. Let your unfailing love and faithfulness always protect me. (Psalm 40:11 NLT)

Prayer: Thank you, Lord, for bringing me through this time of weakness, sickness, and pain. You have remained faithful to me in all the seasons of my life.

Chapter 75

Faith, Questions, and Solace

I can do all things through Christ who strengthens me. Ruth repeated her favorite verse from Philippians 4:13 once again. She gripped the open pages of her Bible, even though she could recite the verse from memory. In a few hours, she faced another round of chemotherapy and desperately needed God's strength and peace.

Throughout the course of her treatment, she not only read the Psalms, but she prayed them over and over, especially when she couldn't put into words the sorrows piercing her heart. With a pen poised in her hand, she underlined verses and passages that seemed to jump off the pages of her Women's Study Bible—Words of life she depended on to get through each day. Words that delivered promises of peace and hope.

Ruth never really asked, "Why, Lord?" But she found comfort and answers to her unasked questions in the Psalms of David. Her soul entered into the cries of his heart as she grappled with questions pertaining to the hardships of life. She clung to his words penned so long ago and yet so relevant today. Even the book of Job provided a strange sense of solace. He had endured so much pain and yet discovered God's unchanging faithfulness.

The prayers of family and friends buoyed her faith. Since her brother was a missionary in Bolivia, prayers poured out on her behalf from all over the world. These prayers anchored her hope and conveyed God's peace.

Ruth witnessed God's hand at work in her life, even in the events that led up to her diagnosis. She felt as though God had prepared her to walk through cancer and chemotherapy. Over time, she understood in an even deeper measure that God was truly with her. This reassurance quelled her need to ask the difficult questions. She learned to wait on the Lord, to trust him, and to delight in him. She experienced his presence and his peace.

I would still have this consolation—my joy in unrelenting pain—
that I had not denied the words of the Holy One. (Job 6:10 NIV)

Prayer: Thank you, Lord, for your nearness to me and your lovingkindness as I walk through the hard places of my life and for giving me comfort and peace.

Chapter 76

A NEW MISSION

"Come on, Ruth, you and your girls love these beauty products. Why don't you become a distributor?" her friend had asked. "You can schedule your parties around work and family. The business is a great way to bring in some extra income. You can work as little or as much as you want. This is a great company. They even give away free booklets to cancer patients filled with all kinds of tips and useful information."

After giving the idea some thought, Ruth had decided that cosmetic parties might be fun, something different from the increasing stress in her nursing job. She joined BeautiControl as a consultant.

Several months later, the doctors diagnosed Ruth with ovarian cancer.

Throughout chemotherapy, she continued her beauty consultant business. She enjoyed these social gatherings that empowered women with confidence. The home parties provided a welcomed distraction from the cancer and its side effects, especially the loss of her hair.

While Ruth demonstrated the skin care products, she recounted her journey through cancer and chemotherapy. Her shining countenance reflected the warmth of her heart as she encouraged other women with her story. She shared makeup tips designed to create eyebrows and eyelashes, filling in the vacant contours. Illness-related skin imperfections disappeared beneath the camouflage of cosmetic secrets.

Ruth delighted in her clients, the invoices, and the boxes of inventory that stocked her home office. Since she'd moved into town, her clients found her home welcoming and easily accessible. Selling products for an organization that supported cancer survivors proved to be a rewarding mission.

Once again, she slipped her wig over her bald head, glanced at her watch, and grabbed her bags. She tossed the bulging cosmetic cases into her car. This was a "good day" in her chemotherapy cycle. Time to party—the BeautiControl way.

> See, I am doing a new thing! Now it springs up; do you not perceive it? (Isaiah 43:19 NIV)

Prayer: Thank you, Lord, for opening my eyes to new adventures. You know what pursuits will bring me life and joy. Help me to use my gifts and abilities to encourage others.

Part 8

Anna: Leukemia

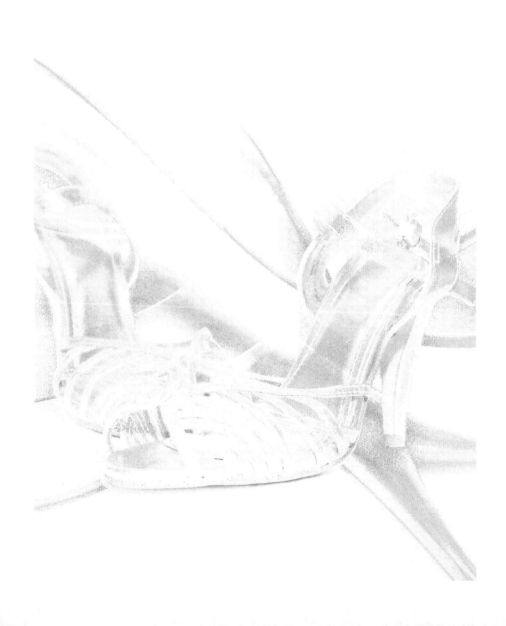

Chapter 77

FACING THE BUCKET LIST

Panting, Anna stopped in the middle of the parking lot to catch her breath. *How can I be so short of breath and tired from just walking from my car into work?* For weeks she suspected something wasn't quite right. Being a nurse, she diagnosed herself. Anemia. As she was busy at home and work, why she might be anemic never occurred to her. All she needed was a blood count and some medication.

She scheduled an appointment at the clinic and left work that Friday intending to be away for about an hour. Unbeknownst to her, she would never return to her job.

After the blood test, the doctor entered the exam room, his lips pursed in a thin line. "Your blood counts reveal that you have leukemia."

Anna sat stunned, unable to process his report in her mind. She was supposed to go right back to work. They didn't even know she was sick.

The doctor continued, "We'll schedule an appointment with the hematologist for this afternoon. Your blood counts are so low that it's even dangerous for you to drive."

How was she going to get home? She'd driven herself there.

While she waited for her appointment with the hematologist, still dazed by the doctor's pronouncement, Anna phoned her husband at work. How was she supposed to tell him she had leukemia?

The hematologist prepped her for a bone marrow biopsy. They needed to determine the type of leukemia so they could administer the proper treatment. After he sedated her, he inserted the needle into her pelvic bone to aspirate a bone marrow sample. She neither felt pain nor remembered the procedure.

After she awakened from the sedation, the doctor returned with the biopsy results. "You have acute myelogenous leukemia, otherwise known as AML. This basically means that the cells which normally fight infection are abnormal. Therefore, your body is unable to resist infection. You have high numbers of leukemia cells and low numbers of healthy blood cells. These cell counts explain why you are so anemic, tired, and short of breath."

Grappling with the ramifications of leukemia, Anna scrambled to dredge up the little nuggets about this disease she had learned in nursing school. Leukemia was not her area of expertise.

When she mentioned the no driving instructions from the other doctor, the hematologist waved his hand and smiled. "Ah, don't worry, your blood counts are going to get much lower than they are now. We'll admit you to the hospital on Monday for chemotherapy. I have to tell you that this is going to be a really rough course, and you may not survive. You may have only a couple of weeks or months to live."

This couldn't be true! She was only fifty-two years old!

Anna stumbled out to her car. She was diagnosed at four o'clock on a Friday. The doctor sent her home for two days of a "normal" life before chemotherapy started on Monday. But life as she knew it careened to a halt.

If she didn't have long to live, how was she going to spend the time she had left? Other people have a bucket list: climb a mountain, fly to Paris, bungee jump. To Anna, these options seemed self-serving. What kind of legacy would she leave? What would she do besides take pills and lie in a hospital bed?

Between breaking the news to her two teenagers, parents, and friends, Anna spent the weekend wandering around her home, numb. There was little else she could do. The doctor instructed her not to engage in any activity that posed a risk of bleeding. He even discouraged the use of sharp knives while cooking.

Anna entered the hospital on Monday morning. Within a couple days, the tests indicated that she didn't have AML, but she had ALL, acute lymphoblastic leukemia.

"Since ALL is normally a childhood cancer, we can't give you a prognosis," the doctor said. "But ALL has a better survival rate, and the chemotherapy regimen is less aggressive."

Unsure of her future, Anna gave up her nursing position. Leaving her co-workers shorthanded for two years while she received chemotherapy would be unfair.

> Let the morning bring me word of your unfailing love, for I have put my trust in you. Show me the way I should go, for to you I entrust my life. (Psalm 143:8 NIV)

Prayer: Lord, I'm so scared to face such imminent mortality. Please help me to trust you with my life and to wisely spend whatever time I have left.

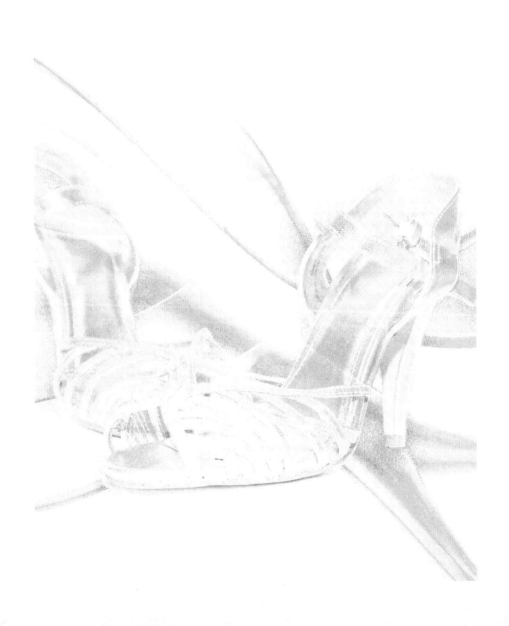

Chapter 78

COMRADES SHORN

Chemotherapy-induced baldness didn't top the list of bad happenings for Anna. Losing her hair paled in comparison to enduring horrendous chemotherapy treatments. The possibility of losing her life tipped the scales. But curiosity niggled at her. What would it be like to lose her hair?

One day in the chemotherapy waiting room, Anna leaned toward her husband. "I wonder what it'll be like when my hair falls out," she said.

From the next couch over, a lady spoke up, "Well, I can tell you what happened to me …"

"I can tell you how hair loss happened with me," another woman interrupted. "My hair gradually fell out, first in clumps, and then my head looked so gross I had to shave it."

Another woman piped up. "One night I went to bed, and when I awoke the following morning, clusters of hair lay strewn all over my pillow."

Their anecdotes answered the questions percolating in Anna's mind. She smiled, grateful for the interrupted private conversation and the candidness of these strangers who encircled her. In the oncology waiting room, camaraderie formed, bonded by a common thread—chemotherapy.

In light of this conversation, Anna clipped her hair short. She abhorred the thought of awakening to discover chunks of hair piled on her pillow or snagged in the teeth of her comb. The wig she purchased proved more bothersome than anticipated. The piece twisted and perched lopsided. Hats provided a more feasible option. Not fashionable hats, but stocking caps to ward off the chill.

Another surprise awaited Anna. No one had told her she would lose every hair on her body.

Perfume and incense bring joy to the heart, and the pleasantness
of a friend springs from their heartfelt advice. (Proverbs 27:9 NIV)

Prayer: Thank you, Lord, for providing me with new friends to help me along this difficult journey.

Chapter 79

LEND ME A VEIN!

Anna guarded her one good vein. When the nurses on her unit were unable to stick the vessel, she contacted her nurse co-workers. With their exceptional skills, they inserted her IV.

Continued difficulty with venous access necessitated the placement of a PICC line, an acronym for *peripherally inserted central catheter*. The doctors performed this procedure for Anna in the radiology department so an X-ray could verify proper placement. She lay on the table, sandwiched between the cold metal and the X-ray machine.

Clothed in gown, gloves, and mask, the radiology resident towered over her.

Giving last-minute instructions, the staff doctor peered over the young man's shoulder, observing his technique as he attempted to place the IV catheter in her arm. Two minutes later, the staff doctor departed. He never returned.

Without offering sedation, the resident jabbed the tender tissue just above the elbow hunting for the prized vein. Soon, numerous pokes transformed into a dig. Trying to hold her arm still, Anna arched her back and scrunched her face in pain. Rivulets of tears welled in her crow's feet and streamed down her cheeks. No one reached out a hand of comfort. No one spoke to her. Finally, the resident successfully threaded the line.

She returned to her hospital room shaking and tearful. As she relayed the tale of this barbarous procedure to her visiting nurse friends, their jaws dropped in shock and outrage. As patient advocates—and even more so for a friend—they complained to the unit manager.

The next morning the head of radiology sauntered into her hospital room and offered an apology.

Too late. Little consolation for all the anguish she had suffered.

> But as for me, afflicted and in pain—may your salvation, God, protect me. (Psalm 69:29 NIV)

Prayer: Lord, help me to remember that no matter what happens, you are with me, and nothing can separate me from the love you have for me. Please help me to forgive those who hurt me.

Chapter 80

Legs Aquiver

Anna wrapped her trembling fingers around the rail. Once again, her husband gripped her arm and hoisted her up the next step. She couldn't raise her foot more than a few inches off the floor, not high enough to climb the stairs in their two-story home. Chemotherapy had siphoned the strength from her leg muscles.

Weakness afflicted not only her legs, but also her upper body. When she could no longer roll over in bed, her husband grasped her shoulders, rolled her to the edge of the bed, and pulled her to a sitting position. Before leaving for work, he slid her pants over her feet and slipped on her socks and shoes.

One day, Anna braced her hands against the armrests of her favorite chair and pushed. She couldn't raise herself up from the seat. Her husband shoved bricks under the chair legs, sofa, and bed. Gripping the arms, she slid forward until her feet touched the floor, enabling her to stand upright. For extra support and balance, she stationed a walker nearby.

Difficulty rising from chairs translated to toilet seats. How was she going to use the toilet? She couldn't be left alone for very long. A raised toilet seat enabled her to slide forward, plant her feet on the floor, and stand.

The tentacles of fatigue extended beyond Anna's home. On a "good" day in the chemotherapy cycle, she and her husband decided to go grocery shopping. As they drove to the store, Anna thought how nice it was to be out of the house for a change.

She remained with the cart while her husband headed down another aisle. The little stamina she'd mustered for the trip had drained. Her legs buckled. She clenched the handle of the cart. Stranded with no accessible phone, she scanned the aisle, searching for a bench. But she spotted only shelves crammed with groceries. Anna broke into a cold sweat, each passing second measured by a quivering muscle fiber.

When her husband returned, he found her crumpled over the grocery cart. He wrapped his arms around her, steadying her as he guided her back to the car.

Anna sank into the seat and closed her eyes. Maybe they'd shop another day.

Have mercy on me, Lord, for I am faint. (Psalm 6:2 NIV)

Prayer: Lord, it's so hard for me to cope with this weakness and fatigue, but I thank you for giving me people, tools, and strategies to help me remain independent.

Chapter 81

HELPFUL HINTS: FATIGUE

1. Plan in advance foods you think you could tolerate while on chemo to avoid cooking when exhausted. Many soups freeze well. Gelatin and puddings are often tolerated.

2. Conserve your energy. Spread your activities throughout the day, taking breaks in between. Don't force yourself to do more than you can handle.

3. Choose activities that are fun for you.

4. Even simple tasks such as bathing and dressing can be exhausting and require rest before engaging in other activities. A shower chair and grab bars may prove helpful.

5. Instead of drying off with a towel after a shower, wrap yourself in a terrycloth bathrobe to conserve energy. Wrap a towel around your head turban style.

6. Spread housekeeping tasks throughout the week. Sit whenever possible and ask for help.

7. Keep in mind that you can purchase many items online, including groceries. Avoid peak shopping times. Make a list. Plan your route in advance to avoid backtracking. Go with someone who can help you if you get too tired.

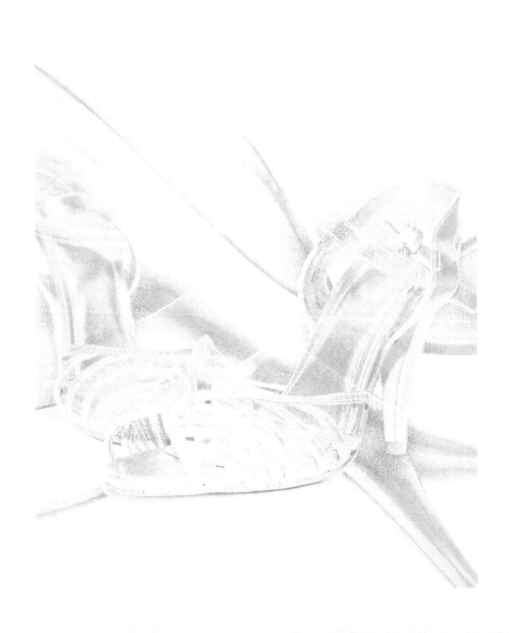

Chapter 82

DRUGS, BUGS, AND BONA FIDE GRIT

Anna's blood counts had dropped dangerously low, placing her at risk for infection. Once again, the hospital staff greeted her clad in their gowns, gloves, and masks. She recognized a strange sense of security in their garb, isolated and protected.

Once discharged from the hospital, she lacked the stamina to frequent the malls, but the isolation didn't prevent her from occasionally going out in public. She donned a mask when her blood counts plummeted, despite feeling conspicuous. She stowed an extra one in her glove compartment. If someone sneezed or coughed in an enclosed elevator, no worry. Her mask protected her from the aerosolized germs. Happiness equaled distance from those germs.

Sources of infection extended beyond people. Though Anna's pet cats delighted her, the doctor was less than enthusiastic with their presence. He instructed her to keep the furry creatures away from her face.

Fresh food also presented an infection risk. The doctor banned all fresh vegetables and fruit, except fruit with washable skins. No plants. No flowers.

Due to the risk of infection, Anna entertained few visitors. Her lack of stamina and muscle weakness thwarted her efforts to shower and then dress in clothing she deemed presentable for company. Besides, if people stopped by, she felt pressured to clean and offer refreshments like coffee and cookies.

Determined to be helpful, Anna's co-workers clicked the computer keys, searching for any medical information related to leukemia. They printed article after article, sending her every scrap of data, every statistic, and any possible thing that could go wrong. Overwhelmed, Anna pushed the papers aside and declined reading the reports. No amount of information changed her situation. She would walk this path one treatment at a time, one day at a time.

Anna endured six months of aggressive chemotherapy followed by one year of maintenance. She cycled through multiple drug regimens: IV and oral as well as injections into her spinal fluid under sedation. Three times a week. Two times a week. Monthly. Daily.

Some said, "You are so brave to do all of this."

Brave? She didn't have a choice if she wanted to live.

Anna maintained meticulous records of new symptoms and medications. Nurses are good at documentation. With so many bottles of pills, so many times a day, she feared mixing them up. She processed the doctor's instructions in the office, but thirty minutes later forgot what he'd said. She was grateful her husband accompanied her to the appointments.

Stress, chemotherapy, and fatigue interfered with her ability to concentrate. Unable to follow the plotlines of movies or TV dramas, Anna preferred game shows. It didn't matter if she forgot the previous question, word, or prize. She could track one game, puzzle, or question for two minutes at a time.

After she completed chemotherapy, each follow-up appointment posed a new threat. *What will the blood counts reveal? What if I get leukemia again?* She questioned every unexplained bruise, bleeding, or pain. *Why is my wrist sore? Where did this bruise come from? I don't remember any injury.* Flashbacks of her ordeal jettisoned her back in time.

After she hit the five-year survival mark, she breathed a sigh of relief. "What do I do, or not do, so the cancer doesn't come back?" she asked her hematologist.

"I don't know," the doctor replied. "Nothing. Since ALL is a childhood leukemia, we don't know what to tell you."

Friends and strangers would say to Anna, "You're too young to be retired."

To avoid a lengthy explanation, she simply smiled. The trial of leukemia was not a season she wished to revisit.

For I know the plans I have for you," says the LORD. "They are plans for good and not for disaster, to give you a future and a hope. (Jeremiah 29:11 NLT)

Prayer: At times I wasn't sure I'd make it through this long season of chemotherapy. Thank you, Lord, for bringing me through and for healing me.

Part 9

Val: Breast Cancer

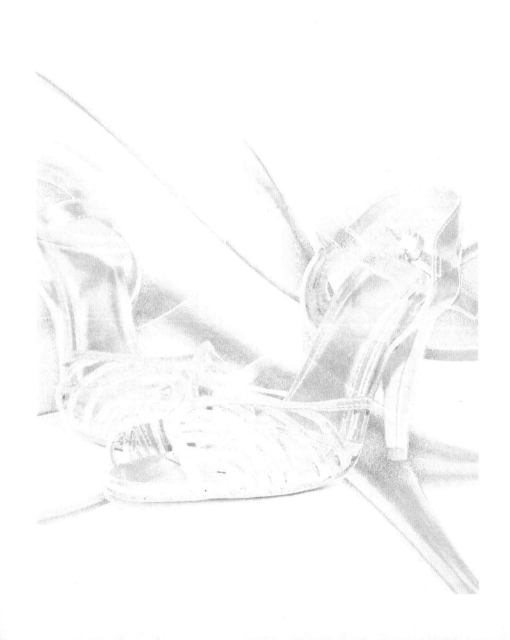

Chapter 83

ONLY A MATTER OF TIME

Val was no stranger to cancer. At eighteen, her high school sweetheart was diagnosed with Hodgkin's lymphoma and underwent surgery and chemotherapy. In her naïveté, it never occurred to her that anyone died from cancer, but her high school sweetheart and future husband passed away at the age of thirty.

She witnessed the agony of her older brother, who slipped away from a cancer that originated in his tooth and grew into a painful facial mass. Twice, breast cancer afflicted her grandmother. Her dad had passed away from esophageal cancer, and at the age of fifty-two, his sister died from breast cancer. Diabetes led to her mother's final demise, despite breast cancer.

"If you had to pick between diabetes and cancer, which would you choose?" Val's sister asked once again.

"Cancer," Val replied. The genes were not good for either one, but her mother's diabetes led to blindness, kidney failure, and dialysis. Val couldn't imagine being tormented with the constant thirst imposed by the restricted fluids on dialysis.

Cancer—it was only a matter of time.

"You got by another year," the doctor said. Val expelled the air pent up in her lungs. Another normal mammogram. With her history of lumps and bumps, she religiously adhered to the yearly mammogram schedule.

While showering three weeks later, she discovered a new lump. Oh no, not another one! After her doctor examined the lump, she scheduled Val for an immediate biopsy.

"Do you think I have cancer?" Val asked.

Her doctor remained silent.

Ignoring the doctor's concerned demeanor, Val wrapped herself in a cloak of denial.

That week, she and her family attended a much-anticipated Kenny Chesney concert. They laughed, stomped their feet, and clapped their hands, but a hazy cloud mingled with the notes from Val's favorite country tunes.

The day after the concert, she arrived at the doctor's office for a biopsy. Since it was Friday, the receptionist handed her a number she could call over the weekend to get her biopsy results. This was a breeze.

That Saturday morning, Val's family left for their various activities, leaving her alone. She refused to allow worry to ruin her weekend, so she grabbed the card with the phone number and dialed.

"You have cancer," the male voice echoed through the phone lines. "If you need any more information, you'll have to speak with your doctor on Monday."

Numb, she hung up the phone. She'd never thought that someone would tell her over the phone that she had cancer.

Val glanced around the empty rooms and then grabbed her jacket. She tramped across the field to her sister's house. Her sister stood in the kitchen chopping vegetables.

"I have breast cancer," Val said.

Her sister cried out, "Oh no!" She whirled around and wrapped Val in a hug. The knife slipped from her sister's hand, and crashed onto the tile floor, barely missing Val's foot.

Val phoned her doctor on Monday. The biopsy results revealed early stage breast cancer. "I'm amazed that you could feel the lump," the doctor said. "The nodule was difficult to find during the biopsy." The doctor referred her to a breast surgeon and an oncologist. Her time had come.

My times are in your hands. (Psalm 31:15 NIV)

Prayer: No matter how I've tried to steel myself for this moment, I'm not prepared to face cancer on my own. Please help me, Lord.

Chapter 84

A Bump in the Road?

Val considered herself a frugal shopper, but the stakes were raised when shopping around for the best breast cancer surgeon. Her surgeon of choice had jockeyed her full schedule and slotted Val and her husband into her five thirty p.m. cancellation.

The anxious couple peered into the waiting room. Empty chairs lined the walls. Val drew in a deep breath and glanced at her husband. Filing past tables littered with magazines, they eased themselves into the side-by-side chairs and waited.

After she finished her surgeries for the day, the doctor strode into the office and took her place behind her desk. She patiently spelled out all of Val's options, which included a mastectomy. Since ductal cancer can hide in other places, she also ordered an MRI.

"I would rather die than go through an MRI," Val said. Memories of panic from claustrophobia while in cars and enclosed rooms boiled beneath her calm demeanor. She shuddered at the thought of being crammed into a tube resembling a large sewer pipe.

Medicated with an anti-anxiety drug, Val climbed onto the MRI cart and lay on her stomach. The technician suspended her breasts into two pockets. She positioned Val's husband at the end of the tube. Reaching forward, Val grasped his hand and clung tightly to him.

"If you can't do this, we'll pull you back out and give you a break," the technician said. "Then we'll try again." The clunks and clamor of jackhammer noises accompanied each cycle, escalating the hammering in Val's heart, despite the medication.

She requested several time-outs before the scan ended. *The worst is over.* Or so she thought.

The MRI didn't reveal any hidden masses, so the surgeon performed a lumpectomy. "The site should fill in with healthy tissue," the doctor said. "You'll probably never even notice a scar."

Good. Six weeks of radiotherapy and she'd be done! A bump in the road.

Several days passed, and Val hadn't received the final pathology report from her lumpectomy. One afternoon, the surgeon called her at work. Val's chest tightened. Something's going on and probably wasn't good.

"We analyzed the tissue pathology," the surgeon said. "You have the beginnings of LCIS, lobular carcinoma in situ. This is not cancer, but there's an increased risk that the breast cancer can migrate to the other breast. Recurrence isn't a matter of if, but when."

Val froze.

"We could just do the radiation for now," the doctor continued. "But under these circumstances, I think the insurance company would pay for a double mastectomy. It's your choice."

"I'll think about my options," Val said with her usual cheery voice. She replaced the phone into the cradle, dropped her head, and sobbed.

That evening, she shared the doctor's report with her husband as they sat huddled together on the picnic table overlooking their wooded lot. In order to avoid further surgery and to ensure a longer life expectancy, they knew that Val had only one option—a double mastectomy.

Clinging to one another, they cried.

> Lord, you are the God who saves me; day and night I cry out to you. (Psalm 88:1 NIV)

Prayer: Lord, I can't believe the news I'm hearing. It's so devastating, and I just don't understand why. Please help me walk through this awful pain.

Chapter 85

THE JUMP TO LIVE

Val stretched her hand toward her husband's, but her fingers slipped through his grip as they wheeled her into surgery for a double mastectomy. Sobs racked her frame. She kept her gaze on her husband, now blurred by her tears. In seven hours, she would awaken to a newly mutilated body. She wanted to live but felt like she was jumping off a cliff in order to save her life.

Still groggy, Val woke in the recovery room. Where was she? Gradually, her vision focused on the wall she faced. Too close. Her stomach tightened. Her hands shook, triggered by the waves of panic from claustrophobia.

Amidst alarms, beeps, and snippets of conversation, she picked up a familiar voice at her bedside. Her surgeon? She was supposed to be doing another surgery. Why was she here? Val's heart monitor chirped in tandem with her rapid heart rate. This wasn't good. Her weighted eyelids spotted the clock suspended on the wall. *That's the clock they'll look at to note my time of death.* Chilled, she tugged the thin blanket around her shoulders.

She never knew what transpired in the recovery room, but eventually the staff rolled her into a hospital room where her family waited.

Determined to go home as soon as possible, Val commandeered her niece, a registered nurse, to help her walk through the antiseptic hallways of the hospital. Her missing breasts unbalanced her center of gravity, and her surgical drains didn't provide an adequate substitute. Numbness in her chest dulled any sensation of pain. But her chest expanders, the first step toward reconstruction, felt foreign and exerted a continuous pressure beneath her skin.

When Val arrived home, she sank into their adjustable bed, and her husband and daughter tucked her in. They'd purchased the bed for her husband's back, but now the mattress conformed perfectly to her exhausted frame. As long as she didn't move, she felt little pain. She could rest and recover in peace.

> Sustain me, my God, according to your promise, and I will live;
> do not let my hopes be dashed. (Psalm 119:116 NIV)

Prayer: Lord, I feel as though I'm jumping off a cliff into a place where I don't want to go, and yet I feel I must take this plunge if I want to live. Please hold me together and help me cope with all of these changes in my body and in my life.

Chapter 86

ON THE ROAD TO RECOVERY

Val avoided peeking at her double mastectomy incisions. Her husband and daughter juggled her dressing changes and emptied her drains between visits from the home health nurse. Only later, while viewing an internet photo, did she realize what her chest probably looked like after surgery.

She arrived home to find that her daughter had created a computerized medication chart and had organized her mom's pharmacy. A friend arranged meals for several weeks. She appreciated all their help, but she also felt humbled, especially since she needed assistance for basic personal care.

Much to her chagrin, she had to forego her makeup. She didn't go anywhere without makeup. She had even determined to wear makeup into surgery, but the surgeon had said no, since they would tape her eyes shut. Eyes taped shut? Just what a claustrophobic person doesn't want to hear.

Along with Val's husband and daughter, a friend engineered a hair-washing soirée. They padded the bed with bath towels and a shower curtain. While Val hung her head over the side of the bed, her entourage dipped a cup into a bucket of comfortably hot water and drizzled it over her thick blonde hair.

Bouts of laughter competed with the splashes of sudsy water that pounded against the sides of the metal tub positioned to capture most of the spillage. As they gathered the slew of towels, the shower curtain, and the tub of frothy water, Val's comrades strutted about in a victory dance. Clean hair with minimal mess and no pain! Tuckered-out, Val would have to wait until morning for her curl and style.

A week after surgery, Val received her pathology report—her lymph nodes looked clear. She let out a huge breath. The report also confirmed that she had made the right decision regarding the double mastectomy. The tissue in both breasts exhibited cancerous changes.

IN HER SHOES: DANCING IN THE SHADOW OF CANCER

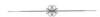

"Beautiful, beautiful!" Val's plastic surgeon said after he removed her bandages and admired his surgical handiwork. She averted her eyes and hoped that one day she could agree. *At least he didn't say, "Oh my!"* She needed to move past the physical discomfort before grieving her loss and dealing with the emotional pain. The surgeon also removed her drains, which she feared would be painful, but they slipped out with less discomfort than ripping off a Band-Aid.

When she finally viewed her scars, she was pleasantly surprised. She wasn't too shocked or upset at the new roadmap that crisscrossed her bare chest. "I know that because of the prayers of my family and friends, I can look at myself and accept my appearance."

The good news continued when Val had her follow-up appointment with the breast surgeon. "You won't need any chemotherapy or radiation," she told Val.

Her activities remained limited, though. She adhered to a thirty-day plan of "no sweating." No laundry, bed making, driving, or raising her arms over her head. She never thought she'd miss laundry or house cleaning. Others scurried about, flushed and glistening in the heat, while she reclined in her chair.

In air-conditioned coolness, she read the plethora of cards from well-wishers. Their enclosed Scriptures and encouraging words brought her comfort and peace.

Val wrote in her blog, "I am reminded that I had forgotten how temporary our bodies are in this lifetime and how wrapped up in this world we become that we forget our purpose in life is to solely serve God."

> "Teacher, which is the greatest commandment in the Law?" Jesus replied: "'Love the Lord your God with all your heart and with all your soul and with all your mind.' This is the first and greatest commandment. And the second is like it: 'Love your neighbor as yourself.'" (Matthew 22:36-39 NIV)

Prayer: I am so grateful for all of those who have shown your love to me during this season. Thank you, Lord, for reminding me that I am here to love you and serve you and to love those you place in my path.

Chapter 87

Fill 'er Up!

"I'm very pleased with how you're progressing," the plastic surgeon said. "We'll start filling those expanders next week."

Val's spirit lifted. The empty expanders that replaced her breasts had flipped, becoming uncomfortable.

Despite her concerns, her first expander filling proved painless. She experienced only a small amount of pressure, since the ports leading into the expanders were located in areas of her chest that remained numb. The first two ounces of saline didn't change her appearance, but every week over the course of two months, the doctors instilled more saline. Since the added pressure in the expanders stretched her chest muscles, they ached for several days.

When Val walked, the saline sloshed, jiggling the hidden sacs. She wrapped her arms around her chest to minimize their movement. Since the expanders pinched and prevented her from sleeping on her stomach or side, sleeping pills provided slumber and preserved her sanity.

The doctor restricted her arm movements and set a ten-pound weight limit. Thankfully, she could play the piano again, but no raking or vacuuming yet—too much arm motion. She probably would never be able to do another push-up. *What a pity.*

Finally, the doctor filled the expanders to capacity. Val joked that he pretended to let her decide the size of her faux breasts. But in the end, the doctor determined expander capacity.

The surgeon removed the temporary expanders and inserted the permanent implants through her mastectomy incisions. She experienced little pain since the mastectomies had deadened the nerves in her chest. Even though the permanent implants felt more comfortable, they still weren't her natural breasts.

Six weeks later, the doctor created nipples in the center of the mounds planted on her chest.

Several months passed before Val was ready for the final step of her reconstruction—tattoos. The surgeon drew a circle around each nipple and injected a local anesthetic. Once again, the numbness worked in her favor. The tiny needles of the tattoo instrument vibrated as they transferred the pigment into her skin, coloring the newly designed areola. At $3000 a side, going to a tattoo parlor would have been cheaper!

Val had been unhappy with her reconstruction, grieving the loss of her breasts, but she experienced something special one day. She pulled out the before pictures of her natural, God-made breasts. *Well, they weren't all that pretty, either.* Even though her newly-reconstructed breasts had no feeling, they actually looked as good as her old ones, in a different sort of way.

"Only God makes you perfect the first time," the doctor said. "We'll never be able to make you perfect, but we do the best we can. You basically traded your breasts for no chemotherapy, no radiation, no Tamoxifen, and no mammograms."

Val was grateful for all that the doctors had done. Her cancer journey had come to an end.

He has made everything beautiful in its time. (Ecclesiastes 3:11 NIV)

Prayer: Lord, this has been a long journey through breast cancer, mastectomies, and reconstruction. Thank you for all those who have helped me along the way and for showing me what's really important.

Chapter 88

RUMBLINGS OF RECURRENCE

"If you find any red bumps on your skin, be sure to come in right away," the doctor had said to Val at her yearly exam. "Since you had breast cancer, you're at a greater risk for skin cancer."

She could no longer brush aside such cautions as she'd done in the past. No longer could she pretend nothing could happen to her. Something had already happened. Fear of recurrence lingered in her mind.

Several years had passed when the doctor noted elevated liver enzymes on Val's blood work. "These labs are most likely a side effect of your cholesterol medication, especially since we increased your dose," the doctor said. "But I know you're worried, so we'll schedule an abdominal ultrasound just to be safe."

The ultrasound technician squirted gel on Val's abdomen and slid the probe across her skin.

Even in the darkened room, she tracked the technician's eyes as they toggled between the probe and the screen.

At various intervals, the technician stopped and made notations: gallbladder, liver, pancreas, stomach.

There are probably tumors everywhere!

Before cancer, Val assumed everything would be fine. But now her thoughts automatically plunged to the worst-case scenarios. If her back hurt, a tumor was probably pressing on her spine. She could never feel quite as secure and unscathed as she did before cancer. Cancer not only changed her life, it changed her perspective.

The day before Thanksgiving, Val received her ultrasound results—normal.

Now, she could truly celebrate with a thankful heart.

You alone, O Lord, will keep me safe. (Psalm 4:8 NLT)

Prayer: Thank you, Lord, that my security doesn't rest on whether or not I have a recurrence, but my security is based on my relationship with you.

Part 10

Pat: Ovarian Cancer

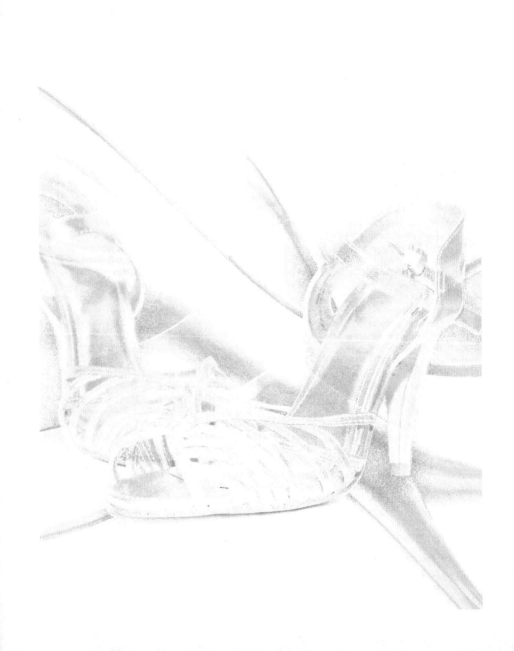

Chapter 89

LEFT IN THE DARK

Pat adjusted the black tiers of her blouse that were cascading over the black-and-white-checked, floor-length skirt. She tried to ignore the gnawing weakness tugging at her left side as she slipped in her earrings. Their feathery tips brushed the matching checked ruffles on her collar and cuff, the latest 1970's fashion. Grabbing her purse and wrap, she joined her husband to travel out of town for his company Christmas party.

She enjoyed the sparkling lights and the festive atmosphere as well as her filet mignon dinner, but as the evening progressed, the weakness pulling at her side escalated. She needed to go home, so they snuck out early.

Pat's regular physician was unavailable, so she scheduled an appointment with his colleague. He performed a pelvic exam and then prescribed an antibiotic for a presumed bladder infection. "If you aren't better in a few days," he said, "come back and see me."

But the weakness persisted.

Several days later, Pat's family doctor examined her. "I feel a mass on the left side of your abdomen," he said. "I think it's your ovary. We need to schedule surgery as soon as possible."

Surgery? Several months back, the surgeon had explored her whole abdomen when he removed her gallbladder. The stresses of the past year whirled about her mind: surgery, three school-age children, neighborhood pranksters bullying her son, and now her mother wintering in Texas.

Pat's surgeon wanted to pursue further testing before the operation. Since the CT scanner wasn't yet available for widespread use at that time, he prepped her for a colonoscopy. After a night of drinking the vile laxative, she knelt on the exam table while he performed the procedure. Without the benefit of sedation, she felt roto-rooted.

Now that the tests were complete, the doctor scheduled Pat's surgery. He never mentioned the possibility of cancer. Besides, Pat was only forty-four years old.

After the operation, the nurses wheeled Pat out of recovery into a room near the nurses' station. IV tubing attached to their respective bottles draped haphazardly around her arms like tangled spaghetti. Flecks of blood clung to the lining of the tubing, the remnants of the five units of blood she'd received in the operating room.

Groggy, she glanced at the clock. Three thirty p.m. Why was she gone so long? They'd transported her into surgery at seven o'clock a.m.

According to her brother, one of Pat's high school classmates had seen the tumor in the operating room and let this morsel of information slip. By evening, rumors that Pat had cancer circulated throughout her small town, providing the main course for dinner conversation. With a wag of the tongue, her diagnosis had spread further than the cancer.

But she remained in the dark.

Night after night, she lay awake huddled beneath the sheets, staring at the clock as the hands ticked down the minutes to daybreak. She strained to hear snatches of conversation from the hushed voices in the hallway, hoping to glean some tidbit of information about her condition. With a quavering voice, she asked the nurses questions, but their answers were vague and skirted around the "C" word.

Occasionally, the night nurses stopped in to chat, interrupting the shadows that danced across her walls. As much as she welcomed their visits, their presence also triggered a disconcerting uneasiness.

No one mentioned cancer.

> Let the one who walks in the dark, who has no light, trust in the name of the Lord and rely on their God. (Isaiah 50:10 NIV)

Prayer: When I feel as though I am left in the dark, remind me, Lord, that you shine your light into my darkness.

Chapter 90

RADIOTHERAPY

The nurses wheeled Pat, IV bags swaying on a pole, to a conference room occupied by her husband and her surgeon.

"We don't have your pathology report back yet, but it looks like you have ovarian cancer," the doctor said to the two of them.

She'd known something was wrong, but she had no idea that she had cancer. She glanced at her husband, hunched over in his chair, silent.

"You'll need radiotherapy to your pelvis and abdomen five days a week for six and a half weeks as an outpatient. Since the tumor spilled over into your abdominal cavity, you'll receive larger-than-normal doses of radiation. The treatments will cause bowel problems which will worsen in the years to come. First, you'll experience diarrhea. Eventually, you'll lose complete control of your bowels."

With tears streaming down her pale cheeks, Pat wrung her hands. She was only forty-four years old. *What about my children?*

Several weeks later, the technician led Pat to the cold metal radiotherapy table. X-rays pinpointed the target area for treatment. With a pen, she marked Pat's abdomen and back. "It's very important you don't wash these marks off until after all of your treatments are completed," she instructed Pat. "We need to target this exact area with each treatment. We'll protect your kidneys and liver with lead shields."

Each day before radiotherapy, Pat had a standing appointment with the local hospital lab. The technician pricked her finger and checked her blood counts to determine if she could receive a treatment that day. When her fingertips smarted as if stung by a swarm of bees, the technicians lanced her ear lobes.

Once she was cleared for treatment, Pat's country club friends drove her twenty-five miles to the University Hospital, even braving ice storms.

Due to the weight of the radiotherapy machines, they were relegated to the basement adjacent to the hospital kitchen. Food aromas wafted into the patient waiting area and triggered bouts of nausea. Odors rankling her nostrils, Pat joined her fellow patients as one by one they clutched their abdomens and entered the single restroom, upchucked, and then dragged themselves back to their seats.

The technician called Pat's name and led her away from the lingering stench of fish, spaghetti, and garlic into a lead-shielded room. She lay on the hard table, sandwiched into position with specially formed molds. Overhead, the radiotherapy machine clicked and whirred like a vacuum cleaner drowning out her voice. "In with the good, out with the bad," she whispered with each breath.

During the forty-five-minute drive home, she threw up every ten minutes. The persistent retching jarred her weakened body. Even on the weekends without treatments, she vomited multiple times a day.

As time progressed, Pat remembered the circle of strangers huddled together in the cramped waiting room united in a common goal—to live. But one by one, the obituary pages in the newspaper recounted the lives of those who bravely endured the treatments and yet lost the battle with cancer.

The side effects of radiotherapy refused to abate even though the treatments were completed. Little by little, Pat relinquished the salads, raw vegetables, and activities she loved. For several years after her radiation treatments, she walked three miles a day and played golf. But the doctors were right. Her bowels moved from diarrhea to loss of control. After several embarrassing accidents, she could no longer stand in line for flights or traverse the golf course. She continued to bowl and play euchre—the restroom just a few steps away.

Such a small price to pay since the doctors hadn't expected her to live.

Surely God is my help; the Lord is the one who sustains me.
(Psalm 54:4 NIV)

Prayer: Lord, sometimes my circumstances are so difficult I wonder if I can still hold on. Thank you, Lord, that when I can't hang on, you hold on to me.

Chapter 91

HELPFUL HINTS: MANAGING DIARRHEA

1. Consult your physician regarding which medications they prefer you to use to manage diarrhea, how much and how often.

2. Drink plenty of fluids, at least six to eight large glasses of water per day or other decaffeinated liquids: broth, Gatorade, or decaffeinated teas. Gelatin and popsicles also offer added liquids. Avoid very cold or very hot fluids.

3. Avoid milk, coffee, alcohol, carbonated drinks, fatty foods, spicy foods, chocolate, raw fruits and vegetables.

4. Avoid high-fiber foods: beans, popcorn, nuts, and high-fiber cereals.

5. Eat smaller more frequent meals consisting of bland foods such as bananas, rice, applesauce, toast, and decaffeinated tea. If you tolerate this diet, then you may be able to add other soft low-fiber foods such as mashed potatoes, white bread, or pasta without sauce, chicken without skin, mild whitefish, canned fruits and vegetables.

6. If you are experiencing anal irritation, you may apply a barrier cream such as Desitin to your anal area. Cleanse the anal area first with warm water and thoroughly dry with a soft cloth.

7. Contact your doctor if you experience any of the following symptoms: dizziness, moderate or severe abdominal cramping or

pain, fever, black or bloody stools, or your medications are not controlling the diarrhea

Chapter 92

RECURRENCE?

Pat clutched her rib cage. With each cough or sneeze, a sharp pain stabbed her side with such ferocity she felt as though her ribs were breaking. She worried that something was wrong with her heart, since she also experienced nausea and swelling in her legs. For two weeks, her physical strength declined until she could no longer get out of bed, prompting her to schedule an appointment with her oncologist.

The doctor prescribed an antacid.

One year had passed since Pat's ovarian cancer surgery. In light of her symptoms, her surgeon also wanted to examine her. He ordered a liver scan.

"There's a mass on your liver," he said. "We think you have cancer."

Even though recurrence lurked in the recesses of her mind, this was not the news Pat expected to hear.

"Because of the effects of radiotherapy on your bowel," the doctor continued, "we're not able to perform any more abdominal surgery. At this point, we have no further treatment options."

She couldn't believe she was hearing this.

The surgeon examined her distended abdomen and decided to biopsy her liver. Pat held her breath, balled her fist and scrunched her face with each stab of the needle. After multiple attempts, the surgeon was unable to snag the necessary tissue samples. Instead, he inserted a needle into her taut belly and tapped off a liter of fluid. He hoped the fluid would reveal the cause of Pat's symptoms as well as provide temporary relief.

How much time do I have left? I'm not ready to die. Who will care for my children? I have to keep going for their sake!

While her husband traveled long hours with his business, Pat shouldered the responsibilities of their home and their children. She staggered through her daily chores: making the beds, washing dishes, cleaning, and laundry, even though some days she struggled to remain upright for more than a few minutes at a time. But she didn't want to burden the children with extra chores. Occasionally, her country club friends stopped by, dropping off a hot-dish, apple pie, or cookies. But food had lost any appeal, which contributed to her debilitated state.

Pat coped by planning daily activities to keep her busy, whether clearing a rabbit's nest out of her rock garden or a trip to the bank. But since they discovered the tumor on her liver, she squirreled herself away in the safety of her home and avoided people, including the church where she sang in the choir. She didn't want anyone to see her cry.

One day, while applying makeup for her weekly outing to the bank, Pat prayed, *Please God, don't let me run into anybody I know.* She feared that if anyone asked, "How are you?" or even spoke to her, the brave face she plastered with makeup might crack and dissolve into a torrent of tears. So far on these excursions, she'd avoided all of her acquaintances.

While at the bank, the mother of a former schoolmate caught her by surprise. "Pat, how are you?"

Pat mumbled, "I'm fine," then spun around and darted into the street as she fought back the tears. *No one must know how bad things are.*

After they had drained the fluid from her belly, she started to feel better. Guarded, she held her breath after each cough or sneeze. But the stabbing pain never returned.

Three months later, the University Hospital acquired its first CT scanner. After Pat's scan, the doctor led her into another room, just as he had previously done when he delivered the ominous news. Her throat tightened, strangling her voice.

With a furrowed brow, the doctor sat across from her. "I've never seen anything like this before," he said as he stroked his chin. "I see no traces of a tumor."

Pat stared at him. *Is he saying what I think he's saying? No tumor?* She drew in a deep breath stretching her vocal cords.

No cancer!

For you, Lord, have delivered me from death, my eyes from tears,
my feet from stumbling, that I may walk before the Lord in the
land of the living. (Psalm 116:8-9 NIV)

Prayer: When illness threatened my life, I felt so scared. Help me, Lord, to cling to you and trust in your goodness and love. Thank you for all the times you protected me even when I was unaware.

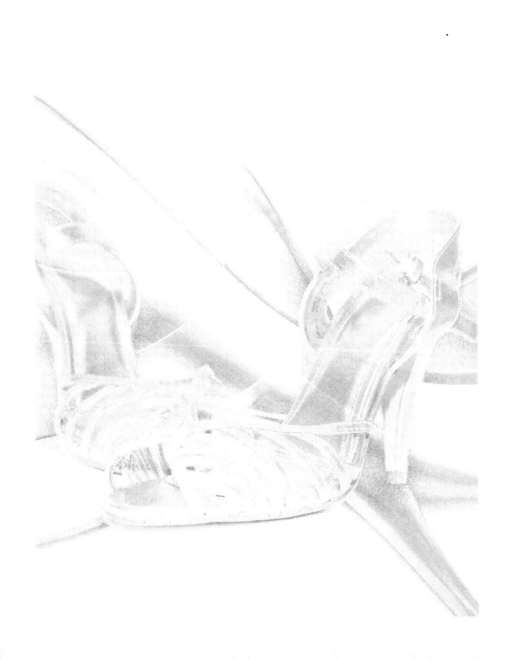

Part 11

Lisa: Brain Tumor

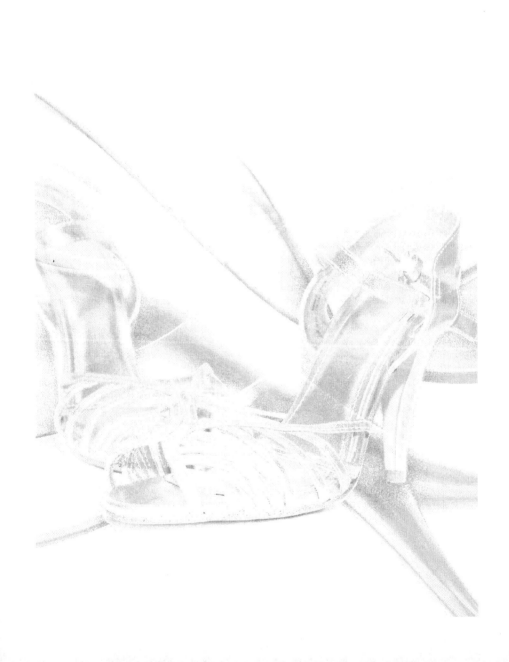

Chapter 93

MIGRAINES?

Lisa massaged her throbbing forehead. Another tension headache. *It's probably just stress.* Even though the pills seemed to offer little relief, she once again popped the over-the-counter pain medication. She resumed packing up her desk and moved to the new office area where the drab walls matched England's overcast skies. Another depressing August day.

For six years, Lisa and her husband worked as US civilians in the Department of Defense, stationed in England. Over Labor Day weekend, they traveled to Rome for a much-needed holiday. During the early morning hours, headaches drummed Lisa awake. The pain medication she gobbled to make it through each day created a rebound effect by thwarting her sleep.

The morning after their return home, Lisa awoke with a pounding headache. Her head throbbed when she bent over, hampering simple tasks such as putting on her socks and shoes. Despite an empty stomach, she vomited. No work today.

By October, Lisa's continual popping of pills matched the raindrops plopping from England's gray skies. Morning migraines accompanied by vomiting greeted her with greater frequency. Occasionally, her left leg tingled and went numb. Since she felt weak and shaky, her husband prepared meals with his chef expertise. Having taken over the driving, he chauffeured her to a doctor, who prescribed migraine medication that included additives to settle her stomach. Because she'd suffered with migraines since childhood, the doctor focused on this diagnosis, excluding any possibility of other causes.

Lisa's physical condition continued to deteriorate. One day, she and her husband left work, ready to leave on a trip to the historic islands of northern Scotland. As they chatted, Lisa's legs buckled. She collapsed onto the pavement.

In lieu of Scotland, she visited the medical center at work, and later that night, the hospital emergency room. The doctors at the medical center checked her blood pressure, eyes, blood sugar, and ran a battery of tests. The results returned normal. Unable to detect anything wrong, the emergency room doctor prescribed sleeping pills.

The next morning, a migraine raged through her head. More vomiting. Lisa asked her husband to drive her to another doctor's office to see the first available physician. When the doctor detected nothing amiss, Lisa requested a CT scan.

The doctor immediately sent a referral to the hospital. "Since you have private insurance, we should be able to schedule your scan in about a week," he said. "Otherwise, it would take three to four weeks to arrange one on the NHS."

Lisa waited, grateful she didn't have the no-cost National Health Service plan offered to British citizens.

Since they cancelled their vacation to Scotland, they decided to drive four hours to a large American military base to be examined at their medical facility. The band of pain had tightened a vise-like grip around her head and refused to succumb to pain medication. A roar like the rush of an ocean's wave battering against the breakers pounded in her ears.

The doctor flicked on his penlight and shined the beam into each eye. "I don't see any indication of swelling in your brain," he said. "Whatever's going on, it's not a brain tumor."

Despite her staggered gait and the increased weakness stemming from her inability to keep food down, the American doctor found nothing wrong. He agreed that a CT scan was a good idea, but since she had scheduled the test in the British medical system, they wouldn't pursue the test any further. He prescribed a new mix of migraine medications, hoping to suppress the headaches from a different chemical angle.

Thankfully, the latest medication offered some relief. Lisa was so tired of popping pills that failed to break the cycle of pain. She blamed the headaches and the subsequent decline of her health on the stress of learning a new job. Maybe the CT scan would provide some answers.

> You are my strength; I wait for you to rescue me, for you, O God,
> are my fortress. (Psalm 59:9 NLT)

Prayer: Lord, I don't know how much longer I can endure this pain. Please help me find some answers.

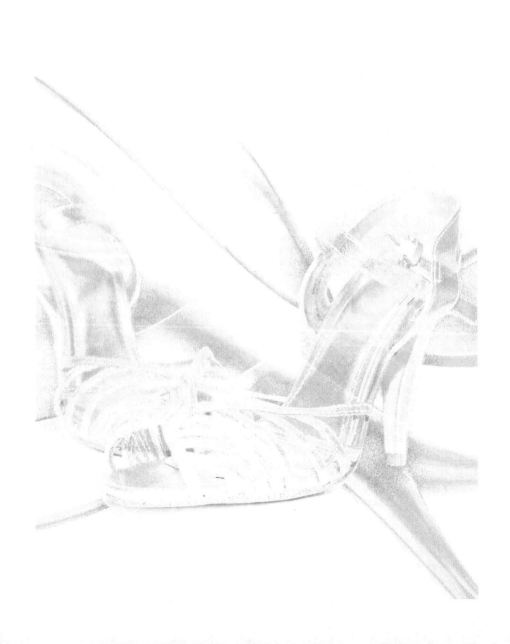

Chapter 94

DESTINATION—HOME

Lisa glanced at the return address on the envelope. She ripped the flap open, pulled out the letter, and scanned the contents. *No!* The doctor had scheduled her CT scan in the middle of their vacation to Italy. She phoned the clinic, and they rescheduled her test prior to their trip.

After the scan, the radiologist sat down with Lisa and her husband. "We spotted an abnormality on your CT scan," he said. "I would like you to see your doctor before you leave on holiday. I've taken the liberty of making an appointment for you tomorrow afternoon."

Something must be terribly wrong.

For twenty-seven hours, Lisa restlessly waited, her stomach knotted.

"It's a good thing you requested a scan," the doctor said. "The CT revealed a cyst above your right eye with some swelling." The report didn't include the actual images of the scan, so the doctor was unable to point out the abnormality. "I'll put you in touch with a neurosurgeon. He'll meet you at the hospital tomorrow evening."

Lisa squirmed in her seat, her insides quivering as they drove an hour to meet with the neurosurgeon.

"You have a cystic glioma, a type of brain tumor," he said. "We aren't sure of the tumor's size, but we need to relieve the swelling and pressure in your brain within the next ten days. We'll know more once we perform surgery and have pathology analyze the tumor samples."

As the doctor scheduled her for surgery, Lisa grabbed her husband's hand.

"I'm also going to prescribe steroids for you to reduce the swelling in your brain and an anti-seizure medication since a brain tumor increases your risk for seizures."

The steroids restored her function to a near-normal level. Her head no longer throbbed. She could even bend over and pull on her own socks and shoes. Despite feeling more chipper, the weeks of debilitating pain, lack of exercise, and poor nutrition had contributed to muscle atrophy. Normally able to juggle multiple activities, even wearying those around her, she now struggled to manage simple tasks.

As the headaches abated, her thoughts turned toward worst-case scenarios. Grasping for answers, Lisa and her husband sought out further medical opinions. The most important decision was whether or not to fly back to the United States for surgery. Lisa's new boss, an old friend, pulled some strings and checked out what kind of care Lisa could receive through the US embassy.

A medical expert from the embassy phoned her. "I've studied your case, and I recommend that you go back to the States immediately," she said. "I'll set up an appointment for you with a neurosurgeon."

Lisa mustered her frayed nerves together and prepared for her departure home, leaving for an indeterminate amount of time. Their vacation destination to Italy transformed into a stateside medical evacuation. Lisa and her husband spent the next two days finishing up paperwork at their jobs and closing up their home for an indefinite period of time. She surveyed the mess, the remnants of their life in England, and collapsed on the bed in tears, shattered and wondering if she could ever pick up the shards.

Neighbors, friends, and church members pitched in and helped them pack, lending not only their hands, but also their support and prayers. God's comfort interrupted their chaos. Their minister prayed with them before their departure. Friends provided a temporary home for their three-year-old miniature schnauzer, Baxter, since Lisa and her husband would be staying with their sponsors in the states during her treatment.

After tearful farewells and hugs, Lisa and her husband boarded a plane for Maryland. Maybe across the sea, they could catch a glimpse of all the autumn colors they'd missed for the past six years, enjoy fresh crab cakes, and reunite with their dear friends and sponsors.

In you, Lord my God, I put my trust. (Psalm 25:1 NIV)

Prayer: Lord, help me to trust in you. I feel so devastated by my diagnosis and all the sudden changes in my life. Please guide me to the right doctors and hospitals.

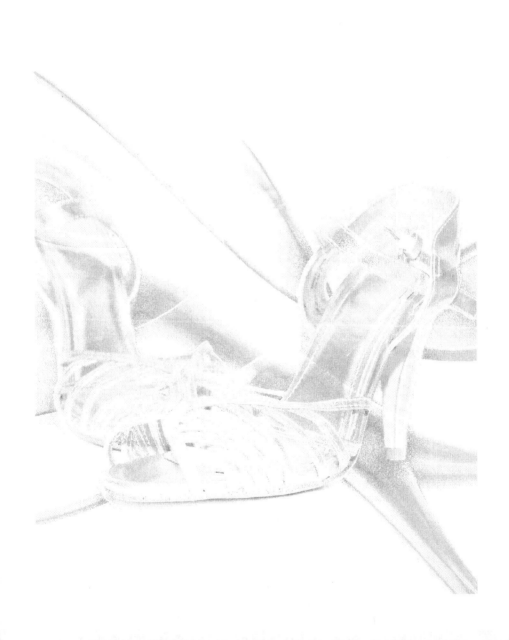

Chapter 95

HURRY UP ... WAIT

Lisa and her husband fidgeted on stiff chairs in the hospital neurology department, succumbing to the exhaustion spawned by sleepless nights, stress, and jet lag from their international flight the previous day. They faced a bank of steel-gray elevators. The doors slid open and closed in tandem to the respective dings as they swallowed and ejected their passengers, the only interruption in their wait for the neurosurgeon.

Two hours later, a staff member approached Lisa. "You might as well get some lunch and come back. The doctor will be a while yet."

After lunch, they returned to their vigil, stationed at the elevator doors. A staff member finally ushered them into an exam room. They perched on another set of rigid chairs, compelling their muscles to hold their bodies upright. Frazzled, Lisa answered the initial script of questions before the technician darted out the door.

She glanced around the sterile room. A chart configured with the human spine hung from the otherwise-bare walls. Once again, they waited.

Twenty minutes later, the surgeon strode in. "In addition to your CT scan, we really need an MRI in order to make the appropriate recommendations," he said. "We'll need to admit you to the hospital so we can perform an emergent scan." Lisa didn't want to be admitted to the hospital, so he set her up for the MRI as an outpatient.

Prodded by lingering fatigue, she combed the MRI waiting room, hunting for a couple of chairs suitable to flop on and catch a nap. She pulled two chairs together, curled up on her makeshift bed, and dozed intermittently.

Four hours later, she stretched out her cramped limbs on the cold MRI table.

The technician positioned a helmet-like coil over her head and instructed her to hold still. Despite earplugs, Lisa cringed, unprepared for jackhammer-style racket interspersed with the clunk of a mallet as the electron particles pulsated and spun, obtaining the appropriate images. She shivered, unable to control her random jerking movements. *Please don't let them have to redo the scan.*

She emerged from the MRI and glanced at the clock—suppertime. They searched for a doctor to review the scan but found none available. Lack of definitive results held her captive in a cycle of fear. Something was wrong but what could it be? And what if she didn't get better?

While in England, Lisa's husband had also contacted another major medical center in the area. They remained in close contact throughout the day.

The next morning, the new neurosurgeon reviewed the MRI, anticipating most of their questions. Sympathetic to the intense emotional gamut Lisa and her husband endured the past few weeks, he agreed that they needed a break. He would schedule her for surgery the following week.

Since the first facility had not yet given their MRI interpretation, Lisa and her husband sought their opinion. They dropped off the scans, but the doctor was unavailable.

Later, he phoned. "I would like to do your surgery today."

That day, Lisa's husband was celebrating a milestone birthday. He didn't need to be sitting in a waiting room on his birthday wringing his hands while his wife was lying unconscious on a surgical table.

Since they felt more comfortable with the second doctor and medical facility, they opted for surgery the following week.

Weary, confused, and scared, Lisa needed a vacation. Her husband booked them into a luxury resort for a weekend of pampering before her surgery. They drank in the autumn colors they'd missed for the past six years. A shower of crimson, orange, and gold leaves splashed across the horizon, replacing the memories of England's fall drizzle.

> The Lord gives his people strength. The Lord blesses them with peace. (Psalm 29:11 NLT)

Prayer: Thank you, Lord, for sustaining us amid our stressful circumstances and strengthening us with refreshing breaks.

Chapter 96

DEBULKED

Upon her return to consciousness after surgery in the neurosurgery intensive care unit, Lisa was immediately assaulted with a throbbing headache.

The medical staff questioned her orientation by asking simple questions. "What is your name?"

"Do you know where you are?"

She mentally surveyed her other faculties for impairments. Her memory and thought processes appeared to be intact. As best as she could tell, her personality seemed unchanged. Except for a little wobbliness, Lisa identified no other impairments, which had been a frightening uncertainty for her when facing three hours of brain surgery.

"We were able to debulk seventy percent of the tumor," the neurosurgeon said. "If the pathology report confirms the low-grade tumor that we detected in the tissue samples, you won't need any chemotherapy or radiation."

Lisa blew out a deep breath and allowed her head to fall back onto the pillow in relief.

Staples crisscrossed Lisa's scalp in a railroad track pattern, forming a pie-shaped wedge. To her delight, she had dodged the doctors shaving her head. Even though vanity violated her Christian principles, she dreaded losing her hair. For days, she scrubbed sticky ointment, rusty orange antiseptic, and dried blood from her hair.

"At least I still have my hair," Lisa said. "Other than a black eye and bangs gelled stiff enough to pose, I look like me."

By the end of the week, Lisa returned home, her skin sporting a collection of holes and bruises in varying shades of purple, blue, and green. She sank into her bed, grateful she would no longer be stabbed, poked, and prodded in the black hours of the night. But even at home, sleep eluded her.

Pain, hospital disruptions, and a body revved up on steroids to prevent brain swelling had interrupted her sleep for weeks. When her exhausted frame finally succumbed to sleep, her husband would wake her to administer medication with a hot chocolate chaser. Once awakened, her mind bolted to the stress of the life-threatening brain tumor and targeted its bull's eye—panic. Her heart raced, and she'd hyperventilate. Coveted sleep was foiled once again.

Despite the lingering weakness and shakiness, Lisa gradually returned to normal, grateful that her mind remained intact. Occasional tightness gripped her head, an expected sequela of surgery since the swelling in her brain hadn't yet decreased.

Her best therapy included the uplifting messages and words of encouragement from friends around the world: England, Italy, Germany, Australia, and Alaska. Humbled and overwhelmed, she felt like Cinderella.

You, Lord, hear the desire of the afflicted; you encourage them, and you listen to their cry. (Psalm 10:17 NIV)

Prayer: Thank you Lord, for providing so many people to encourage me and pray for me during this difficult time. Your love surrounds me.

Chapter 97

The Bubble Bursts

Lisa and her husband arrived at the neurosurgeon's office to receive the final pathology report and treatment plan. They'd been encouraged by the initial report indicating a low-grade tumor, requiring no treatment.

"The final pathology report reveals that the tumor has been upgraded to a grade III cancer, not the low-grade tumor we previously thought," the neurosurgeon said. "These tumors tend to send out spider-like tentacles that are hard to track. I'll refer you to a medical oncologist to discuss chemotherapy as well as a radiation oncologist. I have to tell you that you'll probably lose your hair." He paused. "You also have a third option—no treatment. If the tumor returns, you are healthy enough for us to go back in and surgically debulk the mass."

"The first report seemed too good to be true!" Lisa sobbed.

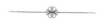

The next week, Lisa scheduled back-to-back appointments with the radiation oncologist and the medical oncologist. Finally, she would be armed with information to replace the imagined scenarios scurrying like rats in the shadows of her mind.

"Your treatment will include six weeks of IMRT, or Intensity-Modulated Radiation Therapy," the radiation oncologist said. "This type of radiotherapy matches the contour of the tumor with laser accuracy and minimizes damage to healthy brain tissue. The appointments will take thirty to forty-five minutes, five days a week, with the actual radiation lasting about ten minutes. You can expect fatigue and hair loss to start at about the two-week mark."

Next, the medical oncologist laid out a chemotherapy plan. "At this point, we can just do the radiation, or we can add six weeks of chemotherapy in a pill form," he said. "This type of chemotherapy is much less toxic than some of the other chemotherapy treatments and doesn't cause hair loss. The most common side effects include reduced blood counts and nausea. We can prescribe some new drugs that are pretty effective in combating the nausea. You can do the chemotherapy during radiation or after the radiation is completed."

Lisa had recently resumed her normal activities and rejoiced in being alive. Thoughts that the treatment would knock her down again delivered a crushing blow.

She mulled over her options and decided to undergo radiation and chemotherapy simultaneously to give the maximum blast to any lingering cancer cells. *If I have to go through six weeks of purgatory, I might as well do the procedures all at once.* Since both treatments would culminate in fatigue, she resigned herself to life as a new caricature—a veggie sprawled on the couch.

Lisa updated her friends in various states and countries, "I'm feeling so wonderfully back to normal right now. Hopefully, I can get through Christmas before I start going downhill from the treatments. Keep those prayers coming."

You make known to me the path of life. (Psalm 16:11a NIV)

Prayer: Lord, I ask you to help me choose the best treatment plan. I trust you will help me through the rough times.

Chapter 98

BRAIN BLAST

The technician positioned a mask over Lisa's face and snapped the device to the hard table on which Lisa lay. "This mask will prevent you from inadvertently moving your head during your treatment," the technician said. "The X's on the mask over the forehead and above each ear mark the sites for the radiation beams. I'll be in the next room operating the machine, but I'll be able to see you on the television screen and talk with you via an intercom system."

Lisa stared at the disc suspended from the arm of the machine, pointing at her head. The arm rotated the disc like the hands of a clock from the eight o'clock position to the ten o'clock, twelve o'clock, two o'clock, and four o'clock positions. As the machine clicked and whirred, the instrument zapped her brain with radiation at each location. A knot formed in Lisa's gut from the chemotherapy pills she'd taken on an empty stomach one hour earlier as instructed. At least she didn't feel nauseated.

Within a couple weeks, Lisa's incision reddened like sunburn from the radiation. She applied a soothing cream recommended by radiotherapy to the divot on her scalp. So far, she managed to hide this bald tract by creatively parting her hair.

One by one, she crossed off the days on the calendar until the end of her treatment. Every day she still had her hair, her energy, and her appetite was a good day.

Lisa established a new daily routine. Since she needed to take her chemotherapy on an empty stomach before treatment, her husband prepared a protein-rich breakfast to carry her through radiotherapy. On the way to the hospital, she stopped at the health club and swam laps. Swimming improved her muscle tone and strength, as well as soothed her frayed nerves. Much to her chagrin, the exercise did little to shed the steroid-induced weight gain.

Clumps of wet hair clung to Lisa's fingers as she combed it out on the way to her treatment. All along the interstate, the wind snatched the flaxen strands from her hand, weaving a trail of silky nesting material waiting to be plucked up by birds. After radiation, Lisa looked forward to her big treat—a gourmet coffee from the hospital's coffee bar, followed by sweet chocolate nibbles.

When she passed the halfway point in her treatment, she felt little cause to celebrate. Radiation had scorched her bangs. The ensuing baldness crept over the top of her scalp and down the sides of her head. At least it was easier to massage the cream into the itchy radiation burns.

Radiation guaranteed several months of no hair growth, so Lisa accumulated a new set of fashionable hats. She'd left her collection of stylish headgear and silk scarves in England. Even though she loved her head coverings, she hoped she wouldn't be chained to an everyday life of caps, hats, and scarves.

As the course of radiotherapy continued, Lisa emerged from her treatments woozy, needing to cling to the doorposts for balance. By sheer determination, she staved off the nausea. She detested feeling ill, taking medications, and dealing with their side effects. A metallic taste lingered in her mouth, which she masked with breath mints and sour candies. Food still tasted good at least.

The subtle effects of the radiation escalated. Lisa questioned whether she could muster the strength to climb the mountain that loomed before her each day. Whether from exercise, radiation, or sleepless nights, a generalized fatigue settled over her like smog.

She was grateful for the social worker at the hospital, her minister, friends, and especially her husband, who propped her up with their encouragement during the course of her treatment.

On a peaceful day, Lisa mused that even though winter had stripped the leaves from the trees, the view from her window was still pretty.

Though the fig tree does not bud and there are no grapes on the vines ... yet I will rejoice in the Lord, I will be joyful in God my

Savior. The Sovereign Lord is my strength. (Habakkuk 3:17-19a NIV)

Prayer: Thank you, Lord, for blessing me with family and friends to help me through the hard places and for giving me strength to get through each day.

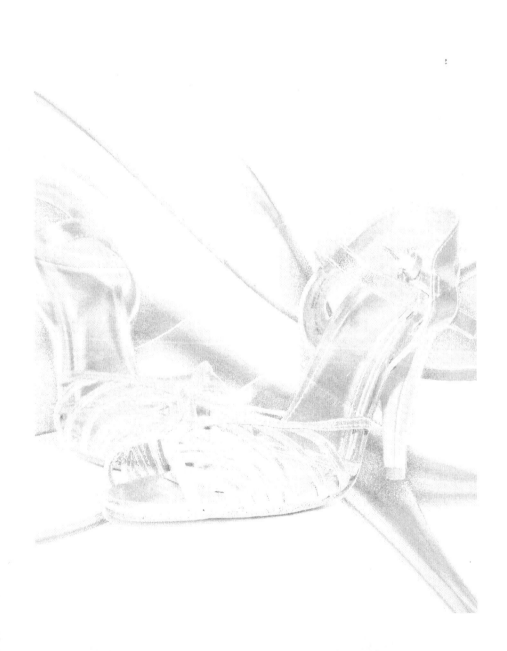

Chapter 99

Helpful Hints: Nutrition

1. Try to maintain good nutritional guidelines.

2. Eat five to six small meals a day.

3. Use liquid or powdered nutritional supplements as needed.

4. Even if you don't feel like eating, continue to drink liquids. Soups and juices can provide valuable nutrients.

5. Chemotherapy may cause food to smell or taste funny. Brushing your teeth and rinsing your mouth several times a day may help.

6. If food tastes too sweet, try sour fruit juices.

7. For foods that taste bitter, add honey or a little sugar.

8. Some foods may have a metallic taste. Avoid canned foods, metal pans, and utensils. Plastic silverware may help.

9. Spices—basil, garlic, onion, oregano, and rosemary—may enhance flavor, as well as lemons, limes, and vinegar.

10. Don't cook your favorite foods while receiving treatment. You may develop an aversion to them.

11. Room temperature foods are often tolerated best.

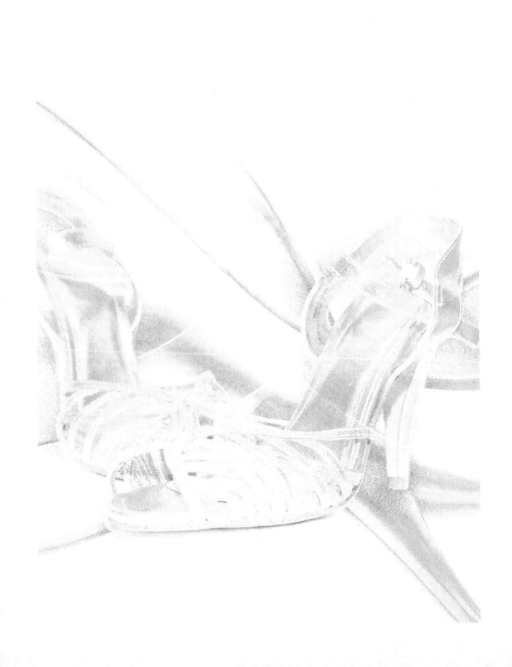

Chapter 100

HIATUS

Four weeks down and two to go. The countdown was on as Lisa's radiotherapy neared completion.

But during one of her treatments, the technician dashed any hopes of a premature celebration. "By the way, Lisa, six weeks of radiation really means six weeks plus three days."

Six weeks was not six weeks and six-tenths! Disgruntled, her heart plunged into a quagmire of despondency. *My doctor's discourteous lack of communication shows a total disregard for me as a patient and as a human being!*

She scrambled to get the chemotherapy pills to cover the three additional treatments. Each day, she struggled to hold herself upright, fighting for the remnants of her strength. Tremors and nausea plagued her ravaged body. Despite a soft pillow, the radiation burn throbbed over her reddened scalp, disrupting precious sleep.

Lisa's scarred head continued to slough clumps of blonde fuzz. Promises of thicker, darker, and curlier hair provided little solace.

When she pointed out to her husband that sixty percent of her scalp mimicked the balding pattern of a male friend, he replied, "But I'm not sleeping with *him!*"

At one point, Lisa had endured enough. She could no longer handle a cancer regimen that destroyed her quality of life. She resolved to quit her treatments and go back to England to live out whatever time remained.

Her husband and the hospital staff intervened, plucking her from the pit of despair, encouraging her to press on.

Thankfully the next day, she felt that the Lord answered her prayers for strength. A new inner peace and calm, which she'd been desperately seeking, surrounded her. She would make it through the remaining medical onslaught.

IN HER SHOES: DANCING IN THE SHADOW OF CANCER

She wrote to her friends. *Please don't think of me as brave, because I'm not. I would love to quit if I could, but I've been thrust into a situation over which I have no control. I'm sure that the reason behind all of this will be revealed to me someday.*

When the radiotherapy center closed over a three-day weekend, Lisa and her husband traveled to a resort for the holiday. The estate, patterned after a French Renaissance castle, rose like a towering fortress between two mountain ranges. A behind-the-scenes tour revealed the ornate opulence of crystal chandeliers, murals, tapestries, and sculpted ceilings. Fine dining included French and Italian cuisine along with a host of culinary delicacies.

While lounging in their luxurious spa, Lisa availed herself of a massage and pedicure. Stress-free relaxation eclipsed the January chill.

Back home, she curled up alongside the crackling flames of a log fire and sipped hot beverages. Between stroking the fur of her canine companions and stitching needlepoint, she marveled at the beauty of the falling snow. Plump white flakes tumbled over one another as they fluttered past her window, until five inches of sparkling puffs blanketed the barren ground.

In the midst of her winter, God had wrapped Lisa in a cloak of love, offering her an oasis of rest.

> Truly my soul finds rest in God; my salvation comes from him.
> (Psalm 62:1 NIV)

Prayer: Lord, you restored my hope and strength, providing places of rest for me even in the midst of this battle for my life. Thank you.

Chapter 101

HOME, SWEET HOME

Home! If all proceeded according to plan, Lisa and her husband would land in England within the week. She anticipated reuniting with friends, not to mention Baxter, their Schnauzer, who would slobber them with his wet doggy kisses.

Their church family and local Bach choir spearheaded a celebration, heralding their arrival in England. But the plans seemed to crumble as obstacles escalated—work releases required by her employer, mounds of medical records to copy, last-minute doctors' appointments, and a New England blizzard.

Her husband collected all her records from the hospital, braving a snowstorm that promised a twelve-inch accumulation. Her fingers and toes cramped from crossing and uncrossing, as she hoped and prayed for no delays. Four months was long enough to be separated from the Bax, friends, and her bed.

The day before her scheduled departure, the medical center called and gave her the medical release she needed to fly to England. Early the next morning, their hostess, a gallant farmer, plowed the snow off the driveway then embraced them through their bulky apparel in farewell hugs. They boarded their flight home despite the fluffy white accumulation.

Lisa and her husband landed in England, but their luggage failed to arrive. Nothing could overshadow the anticipated reunion with Baxter and friends—whether delayed luggage or a driveway dotted with snow, a rare occurrence in northern England. Sunny faces of daffodils flowed over a crystal pitcher and welcomed them into their freshly scrubbed, dusted, and vacuumed home. Their evening meal, ready to be popped into the oven, graced the center of a fully stocked refrigerator and freezer. The overwhelming generosity of friends and co-workers warmed and humbled their hearts.

After a four-hour drive the following day, they retrieved Baxter and joined friends for their homecoming gala. Baxter cuddled on Lisa's lap, refusing to be out of sight of her. Even a little girl tugging on his leash couldn't coax him into a walk. She basked in the sea of happy faces as friends from work, their walking group, their church, and her semiprofessional choir dropped by, wrapped them in hugs and welcomed them home.

The next afternoon, her home fellowship group hosted a tea in honor of Lisa, serving cheese scones, chocolate cake, and fruit breads. Her eyes misted as she sipped tea and chatted with the precious people who made her feel like they'd adopted her as their overseas orphan.

On Sunday morning, an embarrassingly long line of friends embraced Lisa and her husband as they joined in worship at their home church. The cards, prayers, and support from these dear people had often reduced Lisa to tears as she remembered their lovely faces and all the good times they'd shared.

Life returned to normal with Baxter ecstatically frolicking in his own back yard. Her husband returned to work while she unpacked the luggage, amazed at the amount of stuff they'd accumulated after four months stateside. She dumped the bulging suitcases and rifled through their contents in a desperate search for her red beret—a must-have to wear to choir practice that evening. While standing in the midst of the strewn clothes, the doorbell chimed. A dear friend balancing a basket of primroses greeted her. She hastened to gather the clothes, clear a spot for her friend to sit, chat, and sip tea.

Home, sweet home.

> May he give you the desire of your heart and make all your plans succeed. (Psalm 20:4 NIV)

Prayer: Lord, you know the desires of my heart. Thank you for fulfilled hopes and dreams that bring me joy.

Chapter 102

GRAPPLING FOR NORMALCY

Back in England, Lisa's daily routine was not synonymous with life BC—before cancer. Stacks of medical documentation chronicled the tale of her brain tumor and testified to her new life after brain surgery. Everyone she encountered raved about how wonderful she looked, amazed at her normal functional ability. Despite the steroid damage and radiation baldness, she felt reasonably human again and shuddered at the thought of giving up her newfound wellness. She needed a compelling reason to continue chemotherapy at this point.

Lisa juggled medical records and MRI scans as she traipsed into the doctor's office for her first visit with an oncologist in England—recommended by her doctors in the States. She scrutinized the doctor's face as she reviewed her pathology report.

Furrowing her brow, the doctor pressed her lips just like all the other doctors she'd seen.

Each crestfallen gaze crushed Lisa's optimism. She was tired of being lumped into the statistical averages.

Even though the oncologist hadn't had the opportunity to review her records, the doctor offered her medical opinion. "Here in the UK, we normally wouldn't prescribe chemotherapy for a grade III brain tumor like yours. I'm reluctant to continue the chemotherapy since this treatment protocol is reserved for the higher-grade IV tumors ... unless, of course, you insist, and we can prove that you can pay for the drugs with either private insurance or personal funds."

Confused, Lisa fired off an email to her doctors in the States requesting their medical recommendations.

Her stateside oncologist, a leading, world-renowned expert, replied, "There is considerable controversy about how patients with grade III tumors should be managed. Knowing you and your case, stopping chemotherapy now seems reasonable as long as you are followed closely with serial CT scans and careful observation of your clinical status. I'm perfectly comfortable with no further chemotherapy at this point in time."

After the exchange of emails and a second meeting with the UK oncologist, they decided against further chemotherapy treatments.

Lisa rejoiced. Now she could move on.

Back on the home front, she finally arranged to replace their warped and useless patio doors, a repair from the previous year's docket that had been overshadowed by her life-threatening brain tumor.

The workmen arrived mid-morning. When she offered to put the kettle on to brew a proper cup of tea, their eyes lit up, and grins spread across their faces. Plying the workers with cups of tea every few hours seemed to be a prerequisite for making happy workmen, and happy workmen made for a job well done.

Lisa returned to work but lacked the stamina to complete a full shift. She departed for the day when fatigue settled in. Time to lie down and cuddle with the Baxter dog. He didn't mind and clung to her as if he knew something wasn't quite right with his mum.

Lisa emailed her friends. *I'd like to believe that since I'm doing so well and have been spared any tangible loss of function, I stand a better chance than most in beating the statistics. I'm convinced that all of your prayers have resulted in this divine intervention.*

> I particularly urge you to pray so that I may be restored to you soon. (Hebrews 13:19 NIV)

Prayer: I am so grateful for all of the people who've prayed for me. Thank you, Lord, for returning me to my family and friends.

Chapter 103

PRICKLES AND PREDICAMENTS

Once again, Lisa dug her fingernails into the angry crimson rash that raced across the back of her neck, scratching the infuriating itch. She blamed the breakout on the chemicals in the public swimming pool where she regularly swam. But further investigation revealed the rash was a possible side effect from her anti-seizure medication. Despite weaning off the medicine, the burning and itching kept her awake for another miserable night.

Finally, she experienced some relief after her dermatologist prescribed the requested ointments and lotions.

Lisa also met with an epilepsy specialist to discuss the anti-seizure medication she'd been tapering off over the course of the last six weeks. During that time, she battled nausea, fatigue, and shakiness—courtesy of medication withdrawal.

After reviewing her medical records, the doctor shook his head. "I don't understand why you were prescribed such a high dose of this drug without a medication taper," he said. "It's no wonder you've had such a difficult time withdrawing from the medicine. I can also understand your reluctance to try another one."

Two hours later, while working at her desk, Lisa's right hand started to shake. The tremors rippled up her arm into her neck and head. For ten seconds, the seizure clutched the right side of her body and held her captive in its grip. *What's happening? The brain tumor affected the left side of my body, not the right!*

Still shaking on the inside, Lisa left work and phoned the epilepsy specialist. He had departed for a conference, and his backup wouldn't be available until the following morning. Next, she put in a call to the States, but her neurosurgical oncologist was also unavailable and was also attending a conference.

Lisa's general practitioner wouldn't be in the office until the following afternoon. Terrified the uncontrollable shaking would seize her body again, she lay awake all night, her eyes open. She had no medication to treat an epileptic seizure.

She arrived at the specialist's office the following morning to consult with her doctor's partner. Pressed for time, she allowed Lisa a few moments while she rifled through the papers on her desk. "This seizure is probably an isolated episode due to residual scar tissue in the brain from surgery. I'll arrange another appointment for you to see your regular epilepsy specialist as soon as possible." With her gaze still sweeping her desk, she said, "I think you're all right, Lisa."

"As soon as possible" ballooned into a full week before an appointment. Lisa's heart pounded as she vacillated between anger and fear.

Despite the seizure, she was surprised at how wonderful she felt. No bad days, no nausea, and no fatigue. She convinced herself that the seizure resulted from the final hurrah bestowed upon her by the villainous anti-seizure medication. She felt that her body had literally shaken off the last of the medicine from her system.

A few days later, a report on the BBC confirmed Lisa's suspicions—any change in anti-seizure medication, no matter how slight, could trigger seizures.

The epilepsy doctor couldn't identify the cause of the seizure, but he agreed she didn't need a daily anti-seizure medication. Instead, he prescribed a rescue medication to take if she experienced another seizure. The drug would help prevent follow-up attacks.

Two weeks passed without any further seizure activity. Lisa felt like her old self—full of energy, strength, and enthusiasm. She swam a mile in the new village pool, exercised regularly, and resumed her normal work schedule as well as her social activities. She hadn't realized the extensive negative effects of the anti-seizure drug until her body rid itself of the medication's last dregs.

We do not know what to do, but our eyes are on you. (2 Chronicles 20:12 NIV)

Prayer: Sometimes, Lord, I'm scared, and I don't know what to do. Please show me what the right path is for me and calm my fears.

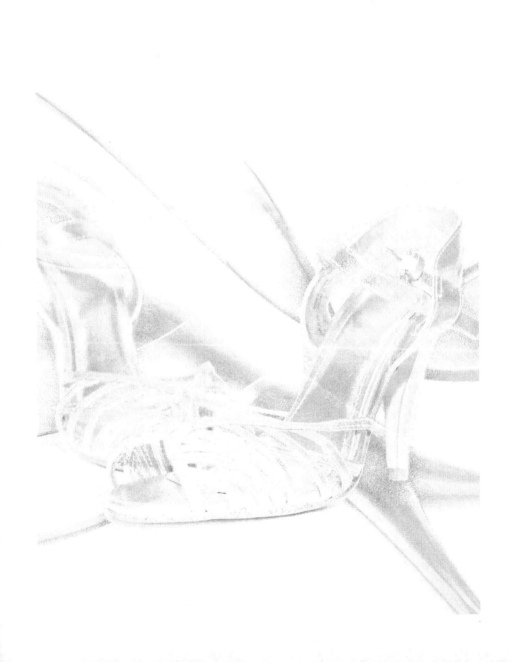

Chapter 104

ANNALS OF THE BALD AND BEAUTIFUL

An unrecognizable hue crept around Lisa's head, refusing to darken the patch targeted by radiation treatments. The shadows of new tufts of hair accentuated the bald sheen wedged front and center on her scalp.

Months might pass before she'd have enough hair to eliminate head coverings. Fragile wisps of hair continued to grow steadily but avoided the turf occupied by the surgical scar.

Spotty hair growth catapulted Lisa into a quandary more dreaded than a bad hair day. Her passport had expired. Herein lay the snag—a new passport required a new photo. Except for religious beliefs, passport photos banned head coverings. Since Lisa abhorred the thought of spending the next ten years flashing a passport that featured a bald woman, her husband printed a passport-formatted picture of her from his computer.

The passport office rejected the photograph. They cited the potential of disguising her appearance by manipulation of the image. Undaunted, Lisa negotiated with the authorities for a temporary passport using the computer-generated photo. She had one year to sprout a full head of hair or purchase a wig before her passport expired. But cancer left a permanent souvenir of her ordeal. Nestled in the surgical divot of her scalp, a palm-sized area of alopecia persisted.

Lisa had always enjoyed hats, especially formal hats deemed unsuitable for everyday wear. However, necessity expanded her millinery tastes to include casual head coverings like berets and newsboy caps. She anchored them fashionably into place with whatever texture of hair she could coax to grow.

Rather than offer strangers the opportunity to gawk at her, she sought out hats to complement her outfits.

A sales clerk complimented her on an aqua pageboy cap while ringing up her purchases. "I wish I could wear hats, but I've never found a style that suited me."

"I never thought I could wear hats every day either," Lisa said. "But once I had to, I found several flattering styles, despite my avoiding them in the past. There's literally a style that will suit every face shape. One just needs the confidence to know what looks right and go with the idea."

> And you shall make hats for them, for glory and beauty. (Exodus 28:40 NKJV)

Prayer: Lord, you bestowed hats of beauty on your priests. I am honored that you have provided beautiful hats for me.

Chapter 105

ANCHOR OF HOPE

In the year since the headaches began pounding Lisa's brow, she traversed continents, health-care systems, a life-threatening illness, and emotional fluctuations. Yet, the suitcases never grew old for Lisa and her husband.

Lisa had completed her chemotherapy and radiation six months earlier, but she still struggled to regain the confidence that she could live a normal life again. "I'm living inside of a body I can't really trust anymore, never knowing from day to day what random symptoms or side effects will crop up," she said. "I have to get used to dealing with these things for the rest of my life. Will they get worse over time, or will they disappear as time goes on?"

Lisa's neuro-oncologist had no answers for her questions or the unexplained phenomena like the transient metallic taste in her mouth that sometimes triggered bouts of nausea.

"We pray the worst part of this nightmare is behind us and that we can now hope, dream, and make plans like any other couple our age," Lisa said.

After enduring nine months of bad-to-mediocre news, Lisa and her husband braced themselves for the next MRI report from the neuro-oncologist.

"There's no trace of cancer," he said.

Tears of joy glistened their smiles. Now they could celebrate.

> We put our hope in the Lord. He is our help and our shield.
> (Psalm 33:20 NLT)

Prayer: Thank you, Lord, for restoring hope and enabling us to dream again.

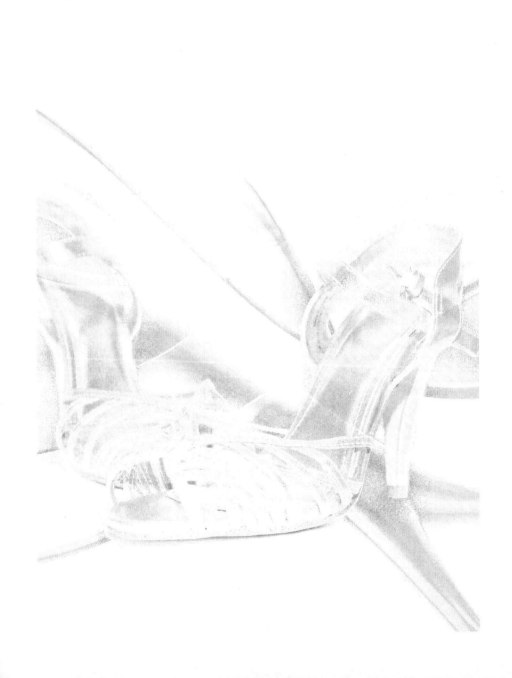

Part 12

Stacy: Breast Cancer

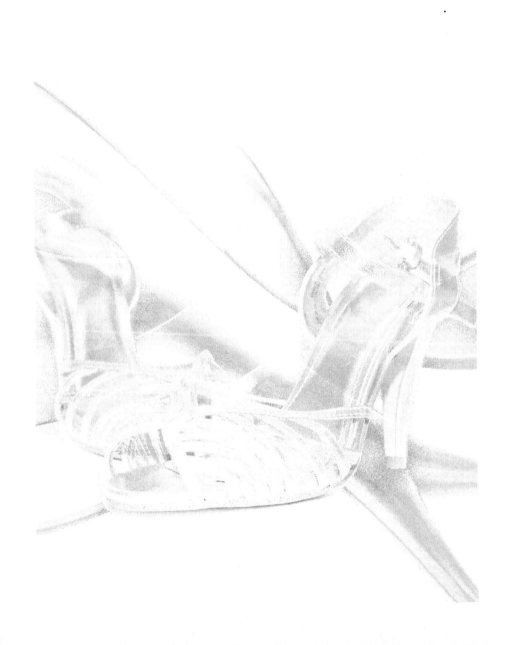

Chapter 106

Daddy's Girl

The nurse poised the wing-tipped needle over her target—the infusaport implanted on Stacy's chest for chemotherapy.

Stacy fainted.

"Stacy, wake up! It's Daddy!"

Daddy—a term of endearment. But Stacy had few childhood memories of her father. He was absent from many family dinners, working long hours as a supervisor on the grain elevators overlooking the international shipping lanes from the Great Lakes, to Puget Sound, to the Mississippi River. He loved the smells of the sea and the massive ships.

Since Dad was now retired, he volunteered to chauffeur Stacy to her four-hour chemotherapy treatments for breast cancer. At first, their conversation choked and sputtered like a car's engine on a cold day, but gradually their nostalgia erected a bridge over the chasm of forgotten memories. Rippling waves of laughter permeated the room as they reminisced.

Dad became a hit with the nurses as he sat by his daughter's side, sporting his golf cap.

Dad and daughter chuckled as they relived the adventures of Al, an orphaned baby alligator caught in the wake of Hurricane Frederick when the storm pummeled Louisiana's gulf coast. Gale-force winds and torrential rains drove the two-foot alligator into a golf course pond adjacent to their home. When hunger pangs struck, Al waddled across the golf course, sidled up to Stacy's sliding glass door, and butted his snout against the panes, foraging for food. Little hands slipped bread and cookies through a slit in the doorway, contributing to Al's eventual eight-foot bulk. After devouring his treats, Al swished his cumbersome tail, turned, and slithered through the manicured driving range back to his pond.

Stacy remembered how her dad had once rescued six baby monkeys from a ship docked at Lake Superior. The antics of the primates tore a path of destruction through their home as those imps ripped the curtains, toppled knick-knacks, and tangled Mom's hair with their nimble fingers. As a result of their transgressions, they were crated and shipped out.

The family braved the world of monkeys again when Dad retrieved an organ grinder's monkey while stationed on the west coast. Charley resided in the basement where he serenaded the family each night with a steady stream of toilet flushing.

One of Stacy's favorite childhood memories occurred on the Fourth of July. That evening, she huddled with her dad in his work tower overlooking Lake Superior. She held her breath, awed by the sparkling fireworks that illuminated the night sky.

But the rocket flares paled in comparison to the fireworks now bursting in Stacy's heart as she unwrapped the gift of her father-daughter relationship. Her ship had come in. She would gladly navigate the rough seas of cancer and chemotherapy all over again just to discover what had been true all along. She was Daddy's girl.

> And we know that all things work together for good to those who love God, to those who are the called according to His purpose. (Romans 8:28 NKJV)

Prayer: Lord, thank you that in your love, you are able to bring good things out of the difficult circumstances in my life. You are my Father, my "Abba, Daddy." Help me to discover the amazing love you have for me.

Chapter 107

TWINS!

Stretching. Bruising. Throbbing. The T-shirt logo "Under Construction" might have portrayed the hidden cataclysmic shifts in Stacy's body. For fourteen months, she anticipated the arrival of her twins—breast implants after a double mastectomy.

Reconstruction plans had rolled out the previous year after Stacy's mammogram revealed a lump in her breast. Three weeks later, the doctor performed a biopsy. The lump had doubled in size. He stroked her arm and apologized in a sweet, hushed tone as he informed her that she had breast cancer. Not having known anyone with cancer, Stacy shrugged. She didn't know why they were making such a big deal out of this. They'd just take that lump out, and she'd be back at her job. Happy forty-fourth birthday, Stacy.

The pathology report revealed a fast-growing cancer. The news burst the bubble that had insulated Stacy from the challenges ahead. Her treatment plan included a mastectomy, chemotherapy, and radiation, all prescribed like a Betty Crocker recipe. She would do whatever the doctor recommended and would press forward unafraid.

While she waited to be wheeled into the operating room, she chatted on her cell phone and smiled and waved as if in a photo shoot. She'd opted for a double mastectomy, which guaranteed identical breasts after reconstruction.

But her doctor had said, "Even the most skillful surgeon can't duplicate God's original design."

Her surgeon reconstructed new breasts by positioning tissue expanders resembling deflated softballs under the skin during her mastectomy. Repeated injections of saline would stretch the skin in order to accommodate the permanent implants, like squeezing into spandex. Another option presented to Stacy involved stretching the abdominal muscles and skin over her chest.

Despite the promised tummy tuck with this procedure, Stacy rolled her eyes as she imagined pregnancy stretch marks crisscrossing her chest like a roadmap.

Stacy laughed and joked after surgery. No tears. With crossed arms, the doctors studied her behavior, seemingly puzzled and alarmed by her cheerful attitude. For four days, they detained her in the hospital, expecting her emotions to plunge like a skydiver without a parachute. They had discounted her upbeat personality.

Every few weeks, Stacy perched on the surgeon's exam table, her fingers curled around the edge. The doctor grasped a palm-sized instrument similar to a stud finder and glided the device over her chest until a point popped up, indicating a metal port. In minutes, he injected saline into the expander through the port. The procedure proved relatively painless since Stacy's chest had remained almost numb since surgery.

Six months after she completed chemotherapy and radiation, Stacy beamed as they wheeled her into the operating room once again. This time the doctor would remove the expanders and insert her implants, complete with a ten-year warranty. Her post-op instructions included consistent massage of the implants to prevent them from hardening, which would necessitate another reconstruction surgery.

She scrunched her face in discomfort as she massaged the firm implants into pliability.

For several months, the implants ached and throbbed, preventing her from sleeping on her tummy. At night, she slid her bottom and shoulders along the curvature of her recliner until she balanced the swollen baseballs mounted like trophies on her chest.

As healing progressed, the doctor completed the finishing touches on the twins. The surgeon clipped a tag of skin from the side of her chest and tacked the section in the middle of the implants to create a nipple. Like a master seamstress, the surgeon sewed dainty stitches in a circular pattern around the newly formed nipple. Eventually this circle would darken, mimicking the areola.

Pleased with her reconstruction, Stacy proudly displayed the twins to her curious women friends. They, as well as her husband, admired her natural-looking contours.

> Again, I will build you, and you shall be rebuilt ... And shall go forth in the dances of those who rejoice. (Jeremiah 31:4 NKJV)

Prayer: Lord, only you can bring good out of my difficult circumstances. You not only rebuilt my life, but you caused me to rejoice again.

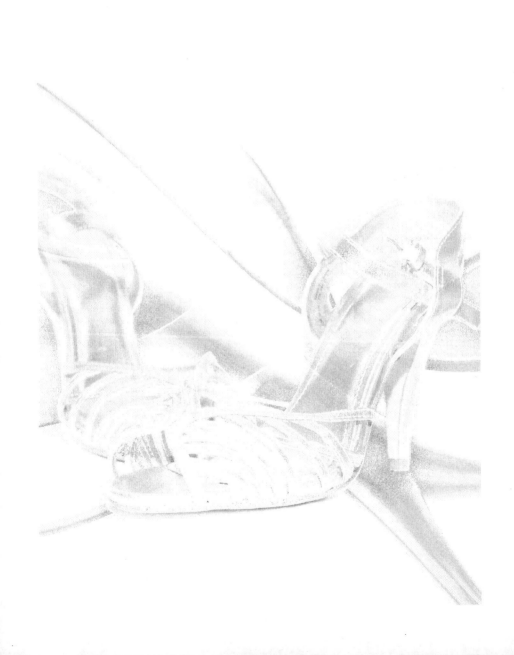

Chapter 108

FIGHT LIKE A GIRL

Knock out Breast Cancer bordered a one-page ad in a local fitness magazine featuring Stacy, a breast cancer survivor. Fuchsia ringlets streaked her new crop of curly, brown hair. Pink lipstick glossed her pursed lips. Clad in a pink T-shirt, Stacy clenched white boxing gloves beneath her chin, poised to strike. Stamped on the boxing gloves—five things a woman should know about mammograms. The fight against breast cancer had evolved into a passion for Stacy.

Stacy had joined a water aerobics class at the YMCA when the aching and numbness in her arm due to the mastectomy limited her arm movements. Impressed with her upbeat attitude, the women in the office labeled her a poster woman for breast cancer survival. When the fitness magazine editors contacted the YMCA, requesting a candidate for a breast cancer awareness photo shoot, they recommended Stacy.

Other gigs appeared on Stacy's schedule promoting breast cancer awareness. The organizers of the Fillies Networking Luncheon requested her to model in their fashion show. The Fillies donated their proceeds to local charities that provided wigs, prostheses, and other services to cancer patients free of charge.

Stacy beamed as she selected a white dress splashed with coral and pink flowers and a matching coral-brimmed hat. While parading across the stage, she sparkled beneath the lights dancing off the crystal chandeliers in the hotel ballroom. She waved to the ladies perched on white linen-draped chairs wrapped with large pink bows as if she were royalty.

When the American Cancer Society announced a Relay for Life in her area, Stacy organized a team. They christened themselves "Team Stacy" because of her contagious enthusiasm. In the first lap of the relay, she joined a sea of purple T-shirts identifying the cancer survivors. Energized by the cheering crowd, Stacy waved and marched shoulder to shoulder with fellow survivors around the track. Then each team member took their turn to walk the track during this all-night event, symbolizing the dark journey through cancer and the teamwork required to overcome the challenge.

Signs cradled by family members tugged at Stacy's heart.

I relay for my mother (or for siblings, grandparents, aunts, uncles).

I relay for more birthdays.

I relay for hope.

A sobering reminder to her of so many lives impacted by cancer.

Darkness fell on the arena and signaled the opening of the Luminaria Ceremony. White candlelit paper bags personalized with pictures and notes lined the track. Each light honored a loved one fighting cancer or a life snuffed out in the battle.

Along with her fellow participants, Stacy walked this lap in silence. Tears pooled in her eyes. So many faces of loved ones dearly missed by their families.

The Fight Back Ceremony, a pledge to stand up and fight cancer through cancer awareness, closed the event. Battling droopy eyelids and muscle fatigue, Stacy rallied along with the other survivors to walk the final lap, branding this pledge upon her heart. Yes, she would take up the fight. She would fight like a girl to knock out cancer.

Be strong and let us fight bravely for our people. (2 Samuel 10:12 NIV)

Prayer: Lord, please give me the strength to continue to fight the battle against cancer, for myself and for others affected by this disease. You alone are our hope.

Chapter 109

SURPRISE!

Stacy collected her purse and Bible, then strode out the door to attend the usual Wednesday evening fellowship dinner, followed by a mid-week church service. As she stepped out of her vehicle, a blast of scorching steam greeted her, threatening to kink her stubby curls. She noticed an unusual number of cars, SUVs, and trucks had converged in the parking lot. *There are a lot of people here for dinner tonight.*

She shoved open the church door.

A chorus of, "Surprise!" jarred her thoughts.

"Oh, my!" Her hand flew to her lips. Beaming faces peeked around pink and white balloons. Pictures plastered the room, depicting Stacy's breast cancer journey—a journey that had drawn her closer to her family and friends, now gathered together to celebrate her forty-fifth birthday and one-year of cancer survival.

With outstretched arms, the children scampered across the room to hug her. A friend draped a pink sash across her chest and crowned her new crop of curly brown hair with a princess tiara.

Pink presents nestled in pink gift bags. The traditional breast cancer ribbon looped the top of her cake.

Her party included those who had dozed on the floor in her hospital room after surgery. Stacy spotted her friend who'd volunteered to drive her to the boutique to select a wig before her hair fell out, comforting her as she wept when the reality of chemotherapy struck her.

And the friend who clipped her hair when bald patches had peppered her scalp beamed at her.

She spied her daughter, who, with a church friend, had presented her with hand-made pink blankets stamped with breast cancer ribbons, which Stacy snuggled into during chemotherapy.

Many had chauffeured her back and forth to her appointments and chemotherapy so her husband wouldn't have to take off work. These champions hadn't allowed her to face this ordeal alone or be the sole possessor of the hospital TV remote.

Memories of the past year flooded Stacy's mind as she scanned the room. She recognized the men who shaved their heads in support of her.

Another guy who frequently bantered with her grinned with a twinkle in his eyes. One day his teasing had backfired.

To get even with him, Stacy had mischievously whipped off her wig. After the initial shock, the church members quickly adjusted to her Wednesday evening attire of large hoop earrings dangling from her shapely bald head. When unable to attend services due to low blood counts, the church had purchased a web cam. Cradled in her recliner at home, she'd enjoyed talking and joking with fellow church members before the service.

In the process, the children had bestowed celebrity status on her. Intrigued by the purple markings on her neck from radiotherapy, the kids asked questions, which she encouraged.

"Why did you lose your hair?"

She explained how she needed chemotherapy, reassuring them that her hair would grow back.

"Can I see your head?"

She had yanked off her wig, and they'd rewarded her with cries of, "Cool!" "There she is!"

Stacy focused to see her pastor approach for a hug. She smiled, the memory of the church's Saints vs. Colts Super Bowl party fresh on her mind. Stacy, the lone Saints fan, had flaunted a black New Orleans Saints baseball cap with a blonde ponytail. During the second quarter, the pastor had promised to wear that hat for a Sunday morning service if the Saints won. True to his word, the next Sunday he preached sporting the Saints cap—the blonde ponytail cascading over his shoulder.

Her breast cancer journey was nearly over. Stacy was so grateful for all the people who had supported, encouraged, and prayed for her, and now celebrated her on her birthday.

And what a relief to see your friendly smile. It is like seeing the face of God! (Genesis 33:10 NLT)

Prayer: Thank you, Lord, for my family and friends who stand by me in my trials—those who pray for me, comfort me, and even surprise me.

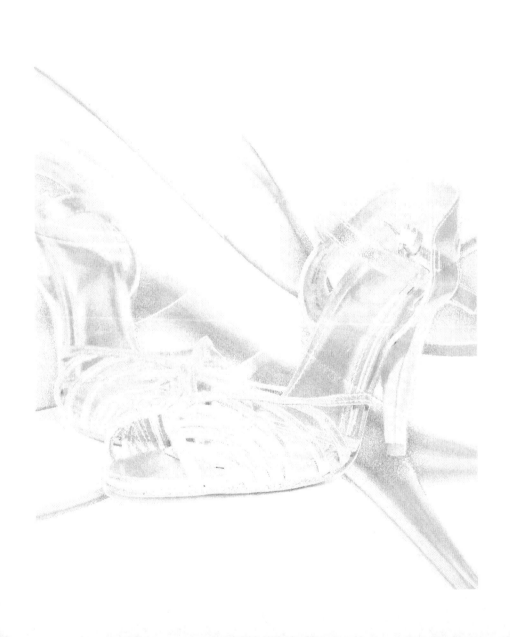

Part 13

Help for the Journey

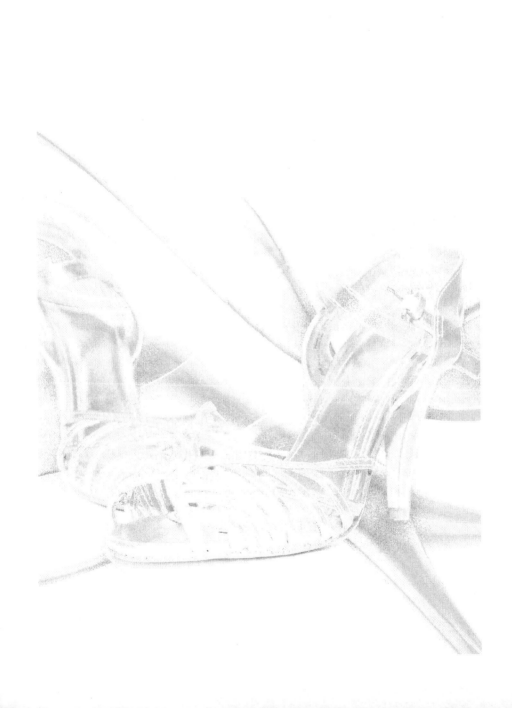

Chapter 110

JOANIE: 12 STEPS TO SPIRITUAL WELLNESS (EVEN DURING ILLNESS)

How do I maintain spiritual wellness when I feel as though my identity and purpose has been derailed by cancer? We are a triune being—spirit, soul, and body—so interrelated that the lack of health and wellness in one part of our being affects the other parts.

For me, spiritual wellness is knowing who I am in Christ and recognizing that he still has a plan and a purpose for my life.

As I called out to God, I discovered the following steps to help restore my spiritual health.

12 Steps to Spiritual Wellness

1. Journaling—I find writing my thoughts, prayers, and feelings helpful as I sort through the plethora of emotions that churn during a health crisis.

2. Scripture—I ask God to reveal to me what verses are relevant to my situation. Then I read and pray these verses, sometimes over and over. I find the Psalms especially comforting as they cover the gamut of my emotional reactions to illness: sadness, loss, depression, betrayal, grief, fear, anxiety, and anger.

3. Prayer and Praise—Prayer and praise help me to focus on who God is. They help me recognize that when I feel like my life is out of control, the God of the universe knows exactly what I'm going through. He understands me, loves me, and has compassion on me.

Prayer doesn't always change my circumstances. But prayer changes me and offers me the ability to cope with my circumstances.

4. Healthy Relationships—My relationships are among the greatest blessings God has given to me. These are the people who have laughed, cried, and prayed with me, and helped me through times of crisis. They've been instrumental in honing my character, forming my identity, and defining my purpose.

5. Rest and Relaxation—When I take time to do the things I enjoy, I feel refreshed, whether I read a book, watch a movie, take up a hobby, listen to music, or play an instrument. I find spending time outdoors invigorates me. I love the warmth of the sun on my face and the gentle breeze. Whether my scenery includes mountains, lakes, wildlife, flowers, or simply the view from a park bench, the wonder of creation reminds me that no matter what's happening in my life, beauty still abounds in my world.

6. Exercise—When I exercise, I need to remember to choose activities within my current physical limitations. I found this out when I attempted to take a short walk and almost didn't make it home. Exercise boosts my mood, helps me sleep better, and increases my energy.

7. Laughter—Whether I peruse *Far Side* cartoon books, watch reruns of *I Love Lucy*, or spend time with funny people, I love to laugh. Laughter releases endorphins and stimulates the immune system. According to Proverbs 17:22, "A happy heart is good medicine and a joyful mind causes healing."

8. Let Go—The phrase for me this year is "Let go!" Let go of anger, bitterness, and resentment—the toxic emotions that drain my energy and strength. Negative emotions suppress our immune systems, and contribute to muscle tension, digestive disorders, stress, depression, and anxiety.

9. Confession—When I confess my sins, I acknowledge that I have made wrong choices. In turn, I receive forgiveness and the opportunity to make right choices. I'm reconciled to God and people, which opens the door to healing from the effects of my sin.

10. Forgive—When I forgive someone who hurt me, my relationship with God is restored, and I release the other person from my wrath and judgment. I love this quote by Marianne Williamson. "Unforgiveness is like drinking poison yourself and waiting for the other person to die." Refusing to forgive another only harms me.

11. Helping Others—When I help others, I reaffirm my sense of purpose. I may not be able to do for others to the extent I was able when I was healthy, but sometimes, a simple phone call, text, or card can bless another person. Doing things for others brings joy, combats depression, and reduces stress.

12. Take a deep breath—A deep breath helps to calm me when I am anxious or stressed. Sometimes I take a deep breath before I open my mouth to speak, so I respond to a conflict rather than react and generate more tension.

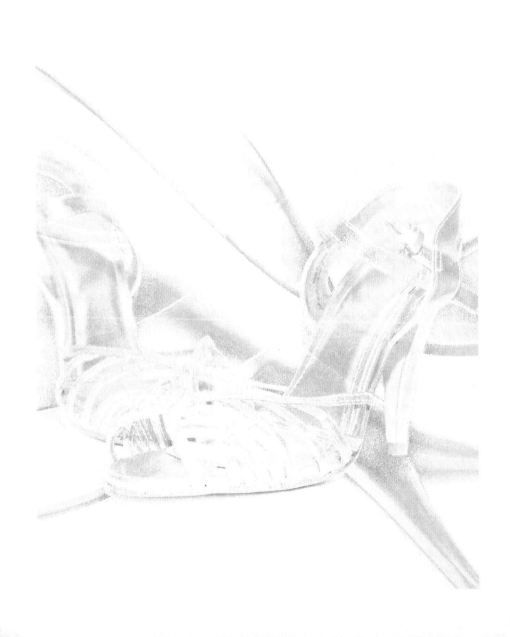

Chapter 111

HELP FOR THE JOURNEY: RESOURCES

The following list is not meant to be a comprehensive list, but provides a starting point for resources:

The American Cancer Society: "Look Good Feel Better" program, wigs and head coverings, specific cancer information. **www.cancer.org**

Gilda's Club: education, support groups (check the website in your local area)

Coping with Cancer Magazine: coping for survivors, caregivers, and medical caregivers. This publication includes educational information and a list of resources as well as stories of hope and encouragement. Available online and as a subscription. **www.copingmag.com**

National Cancer Institute: clinical trials, cancer specific information. **www.cancer.gov**

OncoLink: types of cancer, treatment, coping. **www.oncolink.org**

CaringBridge: free website to connect with family and friends and to keep them posted on your progress. **www.caringbridge.org**

Rest Ministries: support for those with chronic illnesses or pain. **restministries.com**

TLC Catalog: for wigs, head coverings and mastectomy products. **www.tlcdirect.org**

Chapter 112

CONCLUSION: DREAM AGAIN

Nine years after my diagnosis, I had the privilege of joining other ovarian cancer survivors at a camp nestled in the Rocky Mountains near Missoula, Montana—Camp Mak-A-Dream—free of charge for cancer survivors. For some, the camp provided a respite from the ravages of chemotherapy and an unsettling future. For me, it provided an opportunity for new experiences and new friendships with my "teal sisters."

Like many campers before us, we boarded an antiquated school bus and bounced along the winding mountain roads. Amid a sea of teal, the ovarian cancer awareness color, old friends became reacquainted, and new friends were welcomed, all sharing a common bond—ovarian cancer.

We bunked together in cabins that dotted the hillside. After a full day of art, recreation, and classes, we settled on bunks and couches, sharing our cancer stories and offering one another hope and encouragement.

Under the guidance of two gifted artists fighting their own battles with ovarian cancer, we tie-dyed shirts, painted silk scarves, and decorated goodie bags. Throughout the weekend, we tucked little treasures into one another's bags: candy, notes, and ovarian cancer mementos.

Each of us decorated a blank puzzle piece. I embellished my piece with patterned teal paper, ribbon, and letters, spelling out *Fight Girl*. The completed puzzle reminded us that we are connected and do not fight this battle alone.

We hiked, climbed rock walls, balanced on high ropes, and ziplined. On the archery and shooting range, we aimed at our targets and fired. My greatest challenge proved to be the zipline. A staff member encouraged me to step out, despite my terror of heights and fear of injury. She girded me with a helmet and a full-body harness designed to stabilize the spine. I clung to the line, slid off the wooden stand, and sailed over my chasm of fear. The joy reflected in the beaming face of our camp director mirrored my own.

In many ways, the physical challenges paralleled those of cancer: take the plunge, scale the wall, balance, zero in on the target, and shoot. At times, the venture seemed insurmountable, but we celebrated each victory and reminded one another that we are overcomers.

The staff hosted a Super Heroes reception in our honor. Larger-than-life figures of the Incredible Hulk, Batman, Spiderman, Superman, and Wonder Woman lined the dining room. We laughed and posed in our real and imagined superheroes costumes against backdrops of the Hall of Justice, the Heroes Lounge, the Enemy's Lair, and a telephone booth. I joined fellow survivors cloaked in teal as we morphed into caped crusaders fighting our common enemy.

At our closing, we circled together and shared what the weekend had meant to us: new friends who understood the challenges of ovarian cancer, opportunities to try new activities and conquer our fears, strength to press on, hope … and the ability to dream again.

In addition, I connected with other survivors active in the Ovarian Cancer National Alliance. I now share my ovarian cancer journey in the Survivors Teaching Students program, educating medical students about ovarian cancer in hopes of earlier detection.

I'm amazed at the courage of the many women I've met on this journey, the real superheroes who face the challenges of cancer with courage, dignity, and joy.

I hope you've been encouraged and inspired by our stories and that you too will be able to conquer your seemingly insurmountable obstacles and dream again.

It is pleasant to see dreams come true. (Proverbs 13:19 NLT)

Prayer: Lord, I pray that each of these women would discover help, hope, and encouragement in our stories and that you'll enable them to dream again.

Index of Helpful Hints

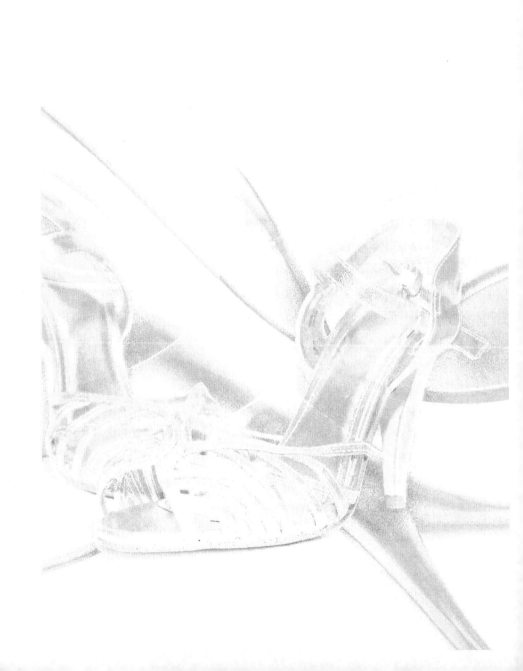

Survivor Notes

Anna retired after her diagnosis of leukemia and enjoys church activities, tying quilts, and reading. She started two book clubs and a coffee klatch.

Cathie has three sons and works for the school system as an assistant superintendent.

Jill swam in college on athletic scholarships. She received a doctorate in educational psychology and is a college professor. She is married with two children

Joanne retired. She enjoys her grandchildren, sailing, and traveling with her husband. After fifteen years with no evidence of disease, she had recurrence and is undergoing chemotherapy.

Lisa and her husband plan to manage a bed and breakfast stateside. When not busy with their twin sons, she enjoys singing in choirs and restoring historical homes. She has experienced recurrence and has undergone surgery and further radiotherapy.

Pat enjoys playing cards with friends. She has had no recurrences. Postscript: Pat passed away November 27, 2018, at the age of eighty-seven.

Rita is married with three sons. She retired from her position as a special education teacher due to recurrence and is undergoing further chemotherapy. Before she retired, she obtained a Master's degree in education. She fulfilled her dream of traveling to Ireland with her husband for their thirtieth wedding anniversary.

Ruth retired and lives near her daughter. She ministers to other women going through cancer by sending cards and care packages and checking up on them through text messages and phone calls.

Stacy is a wife and mother of four. She enjoys spending time with her grandchildren, driving a school bus, and grooming dogs. She loves to inspire other cancer survivors.

Sue is married with two daughters. She enjoys biking, traveling, and cookies. Her rheumatoid arthritis has been in remission since her chemotherapy.

Val enjoys swimming, boating, and spending time with her family. She retired from her position at the local grade school to care for her grandchildren.

And as for me, I was diagnosed with ovarian cancer in 2006 and have had no recurrence. I retired from nursing in 2011. I'm involved in an ovarian cancer social group, The Fried Eggs—Sunny-Side up and speak to medical students about ovarian cancer in the Survivors Teaching Students program. I write articles and encouragement for women undergoing chemotherapy. Publishing credits include *Coping with Cancer Magazine, God Still Meets Needs,* and *The Upper Room.* When not attending one of my two book clubs or my writing critique group, I enjoy designing jewelry, swimming, and knitting.

About the Author

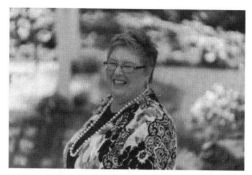

Writer and speaker Joanie Shawhan is an ovarian cancer survivor and a registered nurse. She writes encouraging articles for women undergoing chemotherapy. Publishing credits include *Coping with Cancer* magazine, "God Still Meets Needs" and *The Upper Room*.

Joanie has led small group Bible studies and facilitated Bible-based classes. She has been a speaker as well as retreat planner.

She is a speaker in the Survivors Teaching Students: Saving Women's Lives program sponsored by the OCRA (Ovarian Cancer Research Alliance). Joanie enjoys teaching and sharing her ovarian cancer experience with the medical students. She is an active member in the Wisconsin Ovarian Cancer Alliance and her local ovarian cancer group, The Fried Eggs—Sunny-Side Up.

Joanie has trained under many publishing industry professionals at Write to Publish and the Quad-Cities Christian Writers Conference. She is a member of WordGirls, and a writing critique group, Friends of the Pen. When not writing or attending one of her book clubs, Joanie enjoys swimming, knitting, and designing jewelry.

You may connect with Joanie on her website at www.joanieshawhan.com.

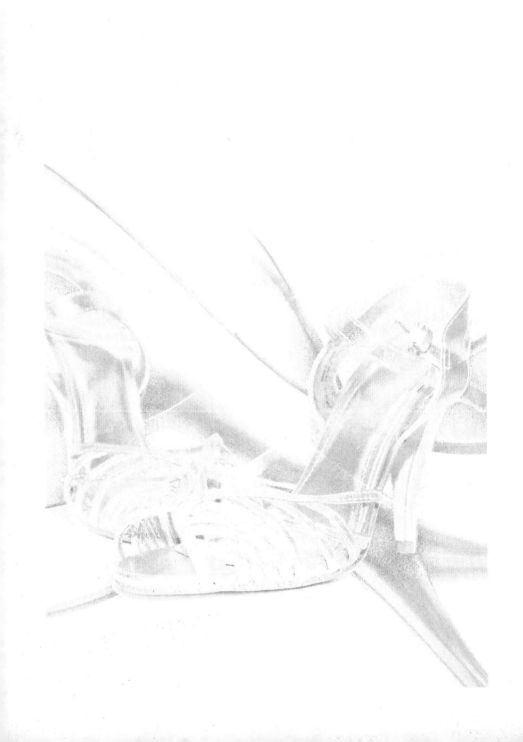